"This is a revolutionary book for **any** woman who thinks she's too heavy. Articulate, entertaining, proud, and unrelenting, **The Invisible Woman** will change our views about fat."

Lindsey Hall
Author of *Full Lives, Self-Esteem Tools,*
and *Bulimia: A Guide to Recovery*

"Thank you, Charisse, for reminding us that a woman's body is not a democracy about which others have the right to vote. No one will be free as long as women must maintain a certain weight and dress size to enjoy basic medical care, civil rights, jobs, and respect. Goodman has used her anger to liberate herself. It's time that we all say 'enough.'"

Margo Maine, Ph.D.
Author of *Father Hunger: Fathers,*
Daughters & Food

"**The Invisible Woman** challenges our most basic assumptions about causes and effects of weight 'problems,' and compares the increasing hatred our society has for large women with the Nazi persecution of the Jews. For all who are terrorized by 'anorexia chic,' and especially for big women who are 'caught in the crossfire between America's cultural conflicts about food and sex,' Goodman makes a passionate plea: 'Let my people go.'"

Russell Marx, M.D.
Director, San Diego Institute for
Eating Disorders

"As Goodman wisely points out, the self-loathing and doubts regarding maturity, will-power, sexuality, and basic worth experienced by millions of women are generated by societal "fattism"—a basic prejudice that, unfortunately, too many of us fail to adequately challenge. Her prescriptions for becoming "visible" once again will hearten and guide those who have been victims."

Joel Yager, M.D.
Professor of Psychiatry
Univ. of New Mexico School of Medicine

THE INVISIBLE WOMAN

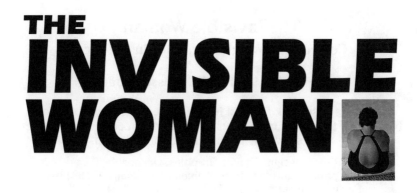

CONFRONTING
WEIGHT PREJUDICE
IN AMERICA

W. Charisse Goodman

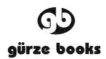

gürze books

The Invisible Woman
Confronting Weight Prejudice in America

Cover design: Abacus Graphics, Oceanside, CA
Cover photo: "untitled" from *Women of Substance* © 1984 by
Patricia Schwarz; PO Box 8084, Berkeley, CA 94707-8084

*Grateful appreciation is given to all publishers for allowing the use of
copyrighted material, as noted within the bibliography.*

Published by:

**Gürze Books
P.O. Box 2238
Carlsbad, CA 92018
(619) 434-7533**

Library of Congress Cataloging-in-Publication Data

Goodman, W. Charisse, 1959-
    The invisible woman : confronting weight prejudice in America / W.
Charisse Goodman.
        p. cm.
    Includes bibliographical references and index.
    ISBN 0-936077-10-7 (alk. paper)
    1. Body image. 2. Overweight women–Psychology. 3. Obesity–
Psychological aspects. 4. Obesity–Social aspects. 5. Sex (Psychology) 6.
Feminine beauty (Aesthetics) 7. Self-esteem in women. I. Title.
BF697.5.B63G67   1995   95-38975
305.9'081–dc20   CIP

2 4 6 8 0 9 7 5 3 1

This book is dedicated to all my friends,
whose humor and humanity make life worth living.

Contents

Author's Introduction

---

*W*hen I look at photographs of myself at the age of four, I see a blonde child of average weight with a sunny, outgoing personality. When I look at the group photograph taken of my kindergarten class one year later, I see the same child with a timid, uncertain smile and lowered gaze who is twice her former size. I see the "baby" of the family who was supposed to remain a baby forever in order to sustain her mother's emotional needs and keep her company. I see a child stuffed with food so that she would never, ever leave home, a child whose mother never wanted her daughter to be her own person or live her own life.

To make things worse, my family moved several times from state to state during my childhood. Not only was I frequently the new kid on the block, but I was always "the fat kid." I wasn't me. I wasn't a name or a person, just an object described by an adjective. If I was naturally shy, I became doubly so. Nevertheless, I learned a lot, and even now, in my thirties, I sometimes wonder if I will ever be able to leave the lessons of my childhood and youth behind completely.

To begin with, I found out early that I'd be lucky to have one or two friends who didn't care what I looked like. I learned that no matter what anyone says, it really doesn't count if you're smart, kind, funny, sweet, generous, or caring because if you also happen to be heavy, you may find yourself on the receiving end of more cruelty than you even knew existed. I learned that keeping to myself and minding my own business didn't help because people would seek me out to ridicule and humiliate me. I learned that "ignoring it," as I was nonchalantly advised to do by my emotionally disengaged parents, usually just made me a greater challenge to bullies, so that I inevitably became "the one to get." I learned that adults are often indifferent to the suffering of a fat child, perhaps because on some level they agree with her tormentors, or maybe it's just convenient for them to believe that an abused child will somehow emerge unscathed into adulthood, magically free of emotional scars.

I discovered that anytime I moved my body, people would laugh at me, and that even if I sat still and quietly read a book they would point and laugh. I learned that if they saw me cry or show any weakness, they would laugh at me even more. And so I learned to cry alone, and laugh alone, and live alone inside my head. I learned that the word "pretty" never included me, and that I was never to dare think of myself or present myself as if it did.

Even those times when I lost weight to try and fit in, it was never enough, and I grew to realize that when it was time to choose teammates for a game, or dates for a dance, I was invisible; but when someone needed a cheap laugh or a quick ego boost at my expense, people saw me, all right. I learned not to go outside because I was afraid to be seen. I learned to walk with my head and eyes down when I had to go out because I knew what I would see in the eyes of others and I knew it would hurt. I learned my place. I tried to learn not to care, and I failed.

I found out that I was condemned, without knowing what I had actually done. I learned that I was not really a girl or, later, a woman; I was a pig, a cow, a hippo, or a dog. I learned that many people take enormous pleasure in hurting others, and they will permit nothing and no one to deprive them of that pleasure. I learned that anyone could harass me with complete impunity, but if I responded angrily in self-defense, I would be scolded for my bad attitude and told that the other kids "didn't mean it" or that they were "just teasing." I learned that self-hatred was my only social right as well as my social obligation.

As I grew up, I assumed a stone-faced mask in order to deprive people of their sickening delight in hurting me, a mask which in later years I would find extremely difficult to remove. I became a tense child with a perpetual air of bewilderment. But I was not angry. Any anger on my part was met by adults with the huffy insistence that I had a hostility problem. What other people did to me was natural and normal, while I was neither.

Now I am a grown woman. I have long made it a point to dress smartly and hold my head up whenever I go out. I don't eat compulsively; nor do I weigh and measure every bite, regret every mouthful of good food. I exercise regularly and moderately. I don't smoke, drink alcohol, abuse drugs, or engage in unsafe sex. Still, everywhere I go, everywhere I look, I must contend with a feeling of invisibility. When I turn on the television, go to the movies, pick up a newspaper or magazine, glance at a billboard, or eavesdrop on the conversations of others, I see and hear the same messages I got as a child. I see one book after another written by experts and laypersons alike who readily, even fervently, reinforce the messages of invisibility. I hear about a survey of North American women in which a majority of the respondents said they feared being fat more than they feared death itself. Worst of all, I know without a doubt that in every town and every city, in every state in America, countless other fat children are learning the same heartbreaking, soul-destroying lessons that I was forced to learn.

In the meantime, it seems that no matter how well I dress, or how intelligent, personable, funny, or caring I am or strive to become, I still must fight to be seen, still struggle for the benefit of the doubt that a conventionally attractive thin woman can achieve merely by showing up, regardless of any personal flaws or internal turmoil. And still, society frowns upon my anger; but there is no longer anything that can hold back a lifetime of rage. My pain and the pain of others like me has been conveniently invisible to thin people for far too long; they have been too comfortable with the price that we have paid for their imaginary superiority. I will neither apologize nor appease. It may not be fashionable anymore, but I don't care; at last, at long last, I am angry.

If you are any kind of fat woman—whether slightly, moderately, or extremely heavy—and you're sick and tired of hearing *ad nauseam* about your flaws, your emotional and/or figure problems, and your allegedly self-destructive behavior, then this book is for you. I don't give a damn about your eating or exercise habits, whether they're "good" or "bad," because the point of this book is that regardless of the state of your physical and emotional health, your so-called excess weight or compulsive habits, NO ONE HAS THE RIGHT TO DISCRIMINATE AGAINST YOU BASED ON YOUR SIZE.

I won't tell you that it's your fault if you're treated like a second-class citizen, or that being fat in America is as easy as being thin if you just hold your head high. I won't interpret other people's prejudice as your low self-esteem when you know you've put your best foot forward. Rather, *The Invisible Woman* is about shattering the stereotypes that have generated the myth of the freakish fat woman. I'm not trying to prove that every big person is a paragon of perfection, civility, beauty, or even good health, but rather that weight prejudice is predicated on the fantasy that the thin person is all of these things, and that therefore any and all harassment and discrimination against the fat person is entirely justified. This book is meant to yank off all the pretty masks that weight bigots use to hide their malice and arrogance from themselves as well as others.

This book will examine, for a change, what precisely is wrong with mainstream American culture and the people who embrace weight prejudice actively or passively—their ignorance, their bottomless terror of becoming fat, and the abuse of the large-sized that often results from that terror. Consequently, a woman who has spent her life loathing fat and projected that loathing onto any woman larger than herself will likely perceive this book as an unfair assault on what she has always considered a universal axiom; likewise for thin people who have a nagging feeling that *something* somewhere in every fat woman's mind or body has gone awry. In fact, *The Invisible Woman* is bound to upset those thin or average-sized individuals who consider their low weight an automatic mark of entitlement if not outright superiority, like the woman in Charles Roy Schroeder's *Fat Is Not A Four-Letter Word* who "told her friends, with a shudder, 'I simply refuse to associate with fat people.'" (Schroeder, 1992, p. 119)

Specifically, this book will discuss weight prejudice as it relates to: (1) health and the prejudice-for-profit weight-loss industry, (2) sexism, (3) the mass media, (4) sexuality, and (5) German Fascist aesthetics and the similarities between anti-Semitism and American anti-fat propaganda. *The Invisible Woman* is intended to be psychological ammunition in black and white, a tool for those of us who know that real prejudice is like a weed with a complicated root system. For the big woman of any age or size who's just beginning to question if weight prejudice is really a natural response to her "problem" or, in fact, a manifestation of other people's problems, I hope this book is helpful. I intend to reveal the subtle and blatant tricks and traps of weight prejudice, and I want to share with the reader the words of some women who refuse to shuffle through life apologizing for their size.

I think the simplest reason for my writing *The Invisible Woman* is that I have always wanted to read a book that says the things I've tried to say here. It's precisely because I've been told all my life to keep quiet, silently swallow abuse, and never bother people with uncomfortable facts or feelings, that as an adult, I feel compelled to point out all the things that people don't want to hear. For instance, no one ever seems to raise the dirty little secret of how thin women, prejudiced or not, for all their body anxiety and insecurities, nevertheless benefit enormously from the exclusive and elitist social games that reward them with opportunities, while fat women, as I've said, often must strive mightily just for the chance to join the game. Female competition—for love, sex, and success—is a topic rarely discussed. As I write this, I'm sitting in a jury room with two TVs both tuned to an interview with none other than Miss America, who perkily explains that the beauty contest provides some of the best scholarship opportunities for American women. What never gets mentioned, naturally, is that no young heavy woman, regardless of her qualifications, ever has or ever will get within light-years of this type of opportunity, or many others like it.

Prejudice, by its very definition, divides people into artificial classes designated as superior or inferior. When racism was at its most powerful in America, white people profited from it in a variety of ways even if they did not support it, while members of other races suffered, relegated to the back seats of the bus and of society. When anti-Semitism was a greater force than it is today, it was Jews who paid the price while Gentiles, prejudiced or not, stepped with relative ease into jobs, neighborhoods, hotels, restaurants, social circles, and country clubs. And now, as anorexic chic fuels the juggernaut of weight prejudice, it is the fat woman, and not her thinner sister, who must endure the contemptuous or shocked up-and-down looks, sometimes disguised and sometimes not, from job interviewers, family members, bosses, co-workers, landlords, friends, dates, and/or lovers or husbands. It is the fat woman who must cope with the smirking or pitying stares from strangers, the condescending and often unsolicited diet and exercise advice, and the substandard medical care from those doctors who scold, threaten, misdiagnose and mistreat based purely on body size. It is the fat woman who must work constantly to like herself despite the braying youths at the swimming pool and beach, the ridicule or disapproving silence when weight lost is regained, the whispers and the wide-eyed gaping if she eats non-dietetic food in public, and the automatic, mindless rejections from men whose faces reflect acute embarrassment or distaste at being stuck on a blind date or at a party talking to a fat woman.

Now, does all this mean that I believe the fantasy our culture feeds us that most or all thin women live lives that are chock-full of unconditional love, success and happiness? Not at all. Does it mean I believe our society cultivates and reinforces a philosophy that thin women *deserve* to live happily ever after? Absolutely. And when enough people truly believe a thing, they will behave accordingly, often resulting in a self-fulfilling prophecy. Thus, the fat woman must conquer the same cultural obstacle that women as a group had to overcome during the early years of feminism; i.e., we often have to break our backs to obtain not only the rights and privileges that others take for granted, but also *the expectation that we deserve them*. And like other groups of people who have fought for equal opportunity, we, too, can overcome, but first we must realize that the problem is bigger, so to speak, than any one of us individually, that it's more than just a question of an insensitive doctor or a rude personnel director, a boss who looks right through you, or a date who checks out your measurements and then keeps checking his watch.

When American women in the early 20th century were told they were too weak-minded to vote, did they attribute this oppression to their own low self-esteem? They did not—at least, not the courageous women who fought for suffrage or supported the cause. When American women were advised that they were not qualified to be police officers, firefighters, doctors, or lawyers—anything besides mothers and housewives—did they rush to therapy to deduct what was wrong with *them* that they should "attract" such shabby treatment? They did not—at least, not the women who could see the problem clearly. It's been said before, and it's worth saying again: the personal is political.

This book is dedicated to every woman who has ever been called a dog or a pig, who has ever been treated as though she were less than female and less than human, just because of her size. The trick mirror that society thrusts before every large woman reflects only society's own panic and misery, and the eyes with which people refuse to see us are clouded by their foolish fantasies. Justice may be blind, but injustice sees only what it wants to see.

CHAPTER ONE

Now You See Her, Now You Don't

The Full-Figured Phantom

---

*There's a rumor, fostered no doubt by the California Chamber of Commerce, that no woman who's short, brunette and fat is allowed to enter California. Brunettes evidently are put into a sealed room at the Los Angeles airport and then shipped back to their city of origin. How else can you explain why **all the women** you see in California are blondes, and long, lithe ones at that, who always swing their hair?*

Lois Wyse
Blonde Beautiful Blonde
(emphasis added)

As bizarre as it may seem, large women in America are to all intents and purposes invisible in today's thinness-obsessed culture, as Ms. Wyse's remark above aptly illustrates. A big woman is neither seen nor heard in our thinness-obsessed society, and is defined purely in terms of her weight and other people's prejudice. Instead of being treated like an authentic human being who just happens to be heavy, she is forcibly transformed by cultural assumptions into an almost mythically unnatural and repulsive figure consumed by physical and emotional problems. Regardless of her unique personal qualities, she is faced with images which portray her as an unattractive, sloppy, even anti-social type. Whatever her individual health habits may be, she must cope with a popular attitude that insists she is compulsive, self-indulgent, sick, and lazy. No matter how well-loved or loving she may be, she constantly gets the message that she is hiding from intimate relationships behind her full flesh. It takes a powerful character not to vanish beneath this avalanche of stereotypes, which is all that American society sees when it looks at a fat woman.

Moreover, most people, despite growing evidence to the contrary, stubbornly cling to the idea that weight is all a matter of willpower. Therefore, the fat woman is perceived alternately as a hostile rebel who just refuses to "get with it" or as a weak-willed slob who doesn't have what it takes to do the right thing. Both attitudes keep the heavy woman at a distance from social normalcy and deprive her of her rightful status as a full-fledged member of American society. Since she is perceived as a type rather than an individual, she is often forced into a marginal existence—on a cultural and/or personal level—as an illusive by-product of other people's conscious or unconscious anxieties, especially if she has been heavy since childhood. All these assumptions, then, combine to create a false image that is so neurotic, unwholesome and unappealing that it is no wonder our perfection-preoccupied society hastens to push out of sight those whom it perceives as ugly losers.

Or does it? Ironically, the invisible woman becomes all too visible—not as a normal human being with normal needs, desires, virtues and vices, but rather as a failure, a buffoon, and an example of what not to be, not to become—when someone goes looking for a scapegoat. Fat people are invariably thrust into the foreground only as anti-role models, when someone decides to make an example of them. Thus, weight bigots such as the playground bully, the insecure thinner person in need of a cheap and easy ego boost, and the producers and promoters of weight-loss products, all see the big woman first and last as a means to their gloating and self-serving ends.

There are many forms of "negative visibility" both subtle and overt. One has merely to glance through any mainstream magazine or newspaper, or turn on the television set, or go to the movies, to observe that not only are large women overwhelmingly underrepresented in the mass media, but also that they are frequently seen as caricatures rather than unique people with diverse experiences. A large woman has only to walk into the nearest shopping mall to realize that the selection of clothes in her size is a fraction of that for thin women, or to note that she must shop in a separate department on a separate floor or in separate stores altogether, where she is out of sight of the "normal" sizes. She need only glance through the average weight-related book to note that society sees her and those like her as permanent "before" pictures, all alike and all in need of salvation. One such work, *The Thin Book,* lists the following qualities as common to "overeaters:" low frustration tolerance, anxiety, grandiosity, wishful thinking, isolation, sensitivity, impulsiveness, defiance and dependence (Westin, 1978).

Like the court jesters of medieval times, big women are typically trotted on-stage solely to amuse and reassure the members of the ruling class. As a result of all these influences, many big women learn at an early age to withdraw into the background to avoid being noticed and battered with negative attention and abuse. Only if the "fatty" loses weight is she permitted to reappear in the foreground of the "normal" world. Only then does society deign to recognize her in a more consistently positive fashion; suddenly, magically, the former failure is visible and validated, and allowed to feel that all good things are both possible and deserved. According to *The Thin Book,* successful dieters possess the following attributes: honesty, willingness, courage, appreciation, open-mindedness, humility, and service (Westin, 1978). Weight-loss testimonials are chock-full of women exclaiming euphorically that their lives have changed: "Now I was slim and [my daughter] wanted to show me off to the world," "I felt like a queen... I looked like a queen," "I am becoming a princess." Humility, indeed. Now you see her, now you don't.

A Day in the Life of a Fat Woman

Dieting is the most potent political sedative in women's history; a quietly mad population is a tractable one.
Naomi Wolf
The Beauty Myth

No one can deny that America is currently in the throes of a gender-specific obsession with thinness, but what does that mean in terms of the quality of everyday life for large women in this country? Let's take a look at an average day in the life of a composite average large lady in an average city.

As she reads the morning newspaper, she sees ads and articles glorifying the slender figure and relegating her own body type to the weight-loss ads. The message: lose weight. You're not a real woman unless you're thin. While taking public transportation to work, she may have to cope with seats designed for much thinner people, some of whom will clearly resent her presence should they have to share a seat with her.

Once at work, she must listen to other women discuss at painful length their diets, their own perceived weight problems, and their anxiety and self-reproach at not being more disciplined. She winces as they express to one another, or her, their disgust and contempt for fatness as a general concept. Eating her meals in the lunchroom results in criticism or comments about her appetite and choice of foods. Perhaps she is even the object of coarse jokes made right to her face, and thinner co-workers who are prejudiced gossip smugly about her. (One man in my former workplace reportedly reacted to news of a relationship between two fellow employees with the immortal words, "That's impossible. She's fat.") She may be discreetly or unconsciously excluded from office or extracurricular social interaction. She may be automatically passed over for promotions, even paid less than thinner people for equal work, solely because her size does not reflect a lean, fashionable corporate image. The message: lose weight. You're not acceptable as you are, and you make us uncomfortable.

Should she have a hairdresser's appointment after work and scan magazines or the salon's catalogues for new hairstyle ideas, she finds few, if any, large women in one volume after another of photographs. Message: your type doesn't belong among pictures of beautiful women. On a clothes-shopping trip, she discovers she must shop in a separate department which is often tucked floors away from the smaller sizes; often she must go to a separate store altogether. When she checks out clothing ads in flyers or newspapers, she finds that garments advertised in sizes ranging from 4-14 or -16 invariably portray a woman at the smaller end of the spectrum modeling the product, and that even clothes for sizes 16 and up may be modeled by thin women.

When she turns on her TV or goes to a movie, she finds a seemingly endless number of slick commercials, programs and plots portraying thin women as attractive, lovable, successful, and glamorous while usually presenting heavy women, when they are included at all, as loud, aggressive, oafish, raw, alienated, etc.; in short, as *un*attractive, *un*lovable, *un*successful, and decidedly *un*glamorous. Practically the only television programming that addresses her directly consists of weight-loss ads. True, sometimes there will be a "special" talk show about large-size fashions or the "special" problems big women face; if she makes enough of an effort, she can even find "special" magazines that actually depict the big woman as normal and attractive, or advertisements for "special" social events or "special" exercise classes geared to large people so they, too, can meet potential mates or exercise in peace. The message? She is set apart from a world that acknowledges only thin people. She is not permitted to "fit in."

Should our lady exercise in public, she will be fortunate indeed if she does not encounter harassment in the form of snickers, pitying or contemptuous looks, or even outright jeering from complete strangers passing by who feel they have every right to comment on her body's size and shape. The irony here, of course, is that weight bigots are quite fond of condemning fat people for their supposed sloth; but when a heavy person does make an effort to engage in exercise, she needs a huge dose of courage and self-confidence to cope with such negative remarks.

Upon arriving home, she may face a companion or family that hounds her about her weight. If she attends parties to try and meet new people, she may find that men are often polite but distracted as they jockey for the attention and favors of thinner, conventionally sexy "babes." Indeed, any public appearance is fraught with unpleasant possibilities.

> Turned away from a city food stamp window because the computer was down, Mara Math had a question: "How are we supposed to eat?" What she heard next from a Dept. of Social Services clerk wasn't much help. "You don't need any more food stamps, honey," the clerk said over a loudspeaker, "you're fat enough already." Jeers and hilarity filled the room. (Roemer, et al., 1993)

What kind of life is this? How much energy do fat women waste just trying to move freely through a world which derides them with impunity purely because of their size, and then insists that unconsciously they really *want* to be abused, that in fact such treatment makes them comfortable because it is familiar? Clearly, our thinness-obsessed society expends a considerable amount of energy to ensure that fat women must struggle just to hold up their heads; moreover, the human misery caused by weight bigotry is expediently attributed to the failures of the fat person, when in fact it stands as an appalling indictment both of modern social values and the American character.

In the chapters to come, we will see that weight prejudice is a true form of bigotry in every sense of the word. Like racism, it is based on visible cues; i.e., the fat person is discriminated against primarily because of the way she looks. Like anti-Semitism, it defines an entire group of people numbering in the millions within a narrow range of negative characteristics and behaviors. Like sexism, it elevates the status of one group of people at the expense of another. And like homophobia, it serves as a vehicle of projection for the bigot's own anxieties, frustrations, and resentments, in effect using the hated outsider as a repository for the bigot's emotional debris and refuse; hence the terms "garbage can" and "dump truck" used to describe the fat woman. In short, weight prejudice is a new twist on a timeless and ugly pattern of human social dynamics.

"Obese and Dirty"
The Damage Stereotypes Do

Why has American culture deliberately chosen to ignore the stereotypes which fuel weight prejudice? Well, at last count the weight-loss industry was raking in approximately $33 billion per year, despite the growing evidence that diets are ineffective and in fact contribute to long-term damage of the heart and the metabolic system. Clearly, encouraging body hatred is extremely lucrative. This obsession with thinness also reveals an irrational but stubbornly-held association between a woman's ability to conform to rigid standards of appearance and her femininity. It deflects attention away from her real accomplishments as a human being—as friend, wife, career woman, artist, lover, mother, etc.—and focuses it instead on her physical characteristics.

*You can have a great personality and be, you know, like
intelligent. But ugly is not going to cut it.*
                                    Male romance game-show
                                    contestant, 1992

In America today, looking good is more than just that, and more
than just feeling good; in the eyes of many, to look good is to *be*
good. Not only are women sent very powerful and relentless
messages that being thin takes precedence over all other goals, but a
woman who is heavy will have to search far and wide for any
mainstream validation of her worth and attractiveness. The mass-
media ringmasters of American society especially convey an attitude
that fat women have no business being in the center ring and should
instead keep to the sideshow with the other freaks. All this is not to
say, though, that big women never achieve love, success, or
happiness, but rather that when they do, it is in spite of today's punitive cultural environment; and when they don't, it is often because
they have been battered since childhood by the pressures of
invisibility.

Millions of women in America wear a size 14 or over. Each is a
unique individual with experiences to match; yet for many, every day
is a silent, uphill struggle for visibility, acceptance, and simple
dignity. If some women continue to put their lives on hold until they
have lost weight, it is because they are bullied into doing so by the
endless cultural propaganda, often reinforced by family and friends,
which tells them they can't truly enjoy life, can't have self-confidence
or high self-esteem, unless and until they are thin. In one weight-loss
book, *Born To Be Slim,* Frank Bruno, Ph.D., goes so far as to
characterize big people who don't want to lose weight and who like
themselves the way they are as "antisocial individuals, also called
sociopaths." Bruno further writes, "The I'm OK position regarding fat
is an unreal position, a position of utter denial" (1978).

There is something deeply disturbing about a culture that insists
on glorifying one extreme physical type while portraying even moderately large women as either neurotic freaks or boring losers. In

fact, in a society of mature individuals, a woman's weight would never evolve into the overheated, hysterical issue that it has become in America; unfortunately, ours is a society caught fast in a state of arrested adolescence. As a result, weight prejudice has evolved into a systemic cultural poison that goes far beyond the routine schoolyard taunting and casual gossip. It can affect the quality of health care a big woman receives or whether she can qualify for— and afford—health insurance. It can be used as an excuse to eliminate her from social and sexual participation or to sever a relationship, and it can mean serious discrimination in the workplace.

> *If I have two equally qualified [people] for employment, one **thin and well-dressed,** the other **obese and dirty**...if I follow this ordinance I have to discriminate against the **thin, clean** one or I go to court.*
> News article about a Santa Cruz,
> California ordinance banning
> appearance-based job and
> housing discrimination;
> Ratner, 1992; (emphasis added)

Comfortable Assumptions

Equally at fault are the millions of women and men who participate in weight prejudice unconsciously and without realizing the suffering they inflict. But conscious or not, there is a certain mindless quality about this form of bias.

For example, big people are frequently accused of being lazy, but the truth is that it is weight bigots, active and passive alike, who are too comfortable with, and too sure of, their superior status to bother examining their assumptions. Blanket statements like "One of the most common unconscious reasons for not losing weight successfully is fear of the opposite sex" (Bockar, 1980) are, in fact, based more upon hackneyed stereotypes than detached psychological research, and completely overlook the individuality of each fat person. Indeed, Dr. Theodore Isaac Rubin's sweeping assertion that "All fat people tend to look alike since fat obliterates distinguishable features" (1970a) sounds suspiciously like the old racist clichés about all black people, Asians, or Jews looking alike. Apparently, Dr. Rubin attempts to nullify fat people's very identities by mentally obliterating their faces.

Another comfortable assumption that contributes to the denial of weight prejudice as a serious matter is that it is at most an anecdotal phenomenon rather than the oppressive institution that it has become. It often seems that thin people are quite willing to admit that fat people are discriminated against, but at the same time seem to think it's something that's taking place quite far away, like famine in Bangladesh or civil war in Africa. Big women know better. Prejudice, like charity, begins at home. I spoke with many heavy women in the process of writing this book, and each one of them, without exception, whether slightly plump or very large, had stories to tell about the disapproval, outright hostility, and arrogant judgments of family, acquaintances, even complete strangers. Comments ranged from loud, harassing remarks made on the street about body size to genuine surprise at seeing a man show affection for his heavy wife or girlfriend. Even mainstream newspaper or magazine articles professing to take a sympathetic tone will describe heavy people in terms one would typically expect from schoolchildren, using words like "fatties" or "tubs"—short for "tubs of lard."

As with other forms of bigotry, it's easy and convenient for those who are not the targets of weight prejudice to consider it a marginal nuisance. However, *The New England Journal of Medicine* pointed out in a 1993 issue that "overweight during adolescence and young adulthood has important social and economic consequences that are more severe for women than for men....obese persons, particularly women, are highly stigmatized in the United States" (Gortmaker, *et al.*).

American society has always been quite content to describe the large woman according to its own demeaning stereotypes. If she says she's not a glutton, the thin world likens her to a lying child. If she says she likes herself "as is," the thin world tells her she's deluded; and if a man insists that he finds her beautiful and lovable, he is likewise dismissed as fooling no one but himself and accorded the same low status as the woman. If she suggests that she could use some breathing room in order to develop in a positive and self-affirming manner, the thin world insists that if she would just get her head on straight and lose weight, she'd be perfectly happy. As one woman who contributed her voice to *Our Bodies, Ourselves* commented:

> One of the difficult things about being large, is that more often than not other people are the problem, not me. Many times I have felt that people I know wonder at my friendship with my lover. They wonder how a thin person can make love to a large one. The idea, I suppose, is that large women aren't attractive. Nonsense, of course. I enjoy my body immensely when I make love, either to myself or my boyfriend. I never think about my largeness. I simply am it and positively luxuriate in it. I love my body when I make love. It is beautiful to me and to my boyfriend. For six years we have both exulted in good lovemaking (1984, p. 187).

The Grand Obsession:
Haunted Women, Wasted Lives

*A cultural fixation on female thinness is not an obsession
about female beauty but an obsession about female
obedience.*

Naomi Wolf
The Beauty Myth

Webster's Dictionary offers the following definitions: "*obsess*: to
haunt or trouble in mind, esp. to an abnormal degree; preoccupy
greatly ... *obsession*: 1. orig, the act of an evil spirit in possessing or
ruling a person... 2. b) such a persistent idea, desire, emotion, etc.,
esp. one that cannot be got rid of by reasoning." (2d Coll. Ed., 1972)

There could be no more apt description of the American
woman's relationship with her body. Possessed by countless images
of perfection always beyond her reach, forever measured and
compared with other bodies, trapped in a world where only one size
fits in, she is truly haunted by our society's grand obsession. Even
when she is acutely aware of the political and social coercion
involved in weight prejudice, she nevertheless finds herself
apologizing for her less-than-"perfect" figure. Whether she conforms
or rebels, she will pay a price.

America's neurotic preoccupation with weight is particularly
ironic in light of the fact that it is the heavy woman who is so often
accused of anxiously interpreting every event and experience in
terms of the food available. In fact, it is the other way around: it is
the weight bigot who zealously scrutinizes every move a big woman
makes through the narrow filter of pounds gained or lost. As a result,
the fat woman is advised that she has certain specific problems just
because she is fat; she must not eat this or drink that just because
she is fat; she is an inferior and burdensome employee just because
she is fat; she is not supposed to think of herself as beautiful just
because she is fat; she obviously has the wrong attitudes about food,
love, and life, since otherwise she would take all necessary steps to

stop being fat; no one loves her just because she is fat, etc. For the weight bigot and the weight-obsessed, thinness is like winning: it isn't everything, it's the *only* thing. It is society's fixation upon weight that poses the greatest threat to the everyday well-being of the big woman.

Obsession is pressure, pure and simple, whether internal or external. If we as a nation are obsessed with thinness—and I have yet to encounter anyone who disagrees with that statement—then it's safe to say that thinness has acquired a highly exaggerated status in assessing a woman's value. Obsession by its very definition is an expression of imbalance and disturbance.

> ***Successful dieting is the most difficult thing you have done in your life or ever will do.*** *If you think you've had some hard times with money, jobs, illness, the death of loved ones, children, school, moving, or getting rejected socially, they are nothing compared to successful dieting....Even the death of a loved one is something you eventually get over and accept to some degree. Dieting goes on (intermittently) forever.*
>
> Joyce Bockar
> *The Last Best Diet Book,* 1980

One of the most curious contradictions of weight obsession is that if a woman succumbs to it and keeps her weight unnaturally low by even the most desperate means, she is popularly considered in our culture to be an attractive person who "cares about herself," even if she risks her health in the process. On the other hand, a heavy woman who shuns this mania and refuses to waste her life fixated on her figure is characterized as unattractive and lacking in self-regard, even as someone who has lost interest in pleasing a mate. "Letting yourself go is an unkindness to your lover, and it's a risky business," one thin female writer wrote in a column about weight gain and romance (Lara, 1991). Once again, the large woman vanishes into the cultural background while the slender woman is promoted as a model of feminine success. The irony is bitter indeed given that weight control, in theory, is supposed to be all about well-balanced health habits. In practice, nothing could be further from the truth.

> *When I saw the picture of Karen Carpenter just before she died [of anorexia], I was thinking to myself, How can I walk that fine line between life and death and still be that thin? How can I get that thin without dying?*
> Christine Alt, large-size model speaking of her bout with self-starvation (Vicki Lawrence talk show, 1994)

The truth is, when people talk about weight and women in this day and age they are not really talking about food or eating habits at all; they are not even talking about health. Weight is really a framework for issues like power, entitlement, control, conformity, and the ways in which society grants or withholds approval, love, sex, social status, and opportunities. This is why weight is such a volatile subject among women. Many are desperate to conform to extreme standards and few have the courage required to change them.

Still, advocates of the weight-loss propaganda machine would like big women especially to believe that this obsessiveness is right and proper, that narcissism and permanent anxiety are not too great a price to pay along with the money spent on dieting, if in the end they transform themselves into thin women. Back in the Twiggy era, diet-book authors Ann Gold and Sara Welles Briller wrote, "you have to hate yourself *enough*" to be motivated to lose weight; they also used phrases like "ugly fat" no fewer than nineteen times throughout their narrative (1968). We have not come a long way since then. In fact, the reader will see in the chapters to come that even quotes from the 1960's and 1970's are still relevant today, since there has been woefully little progress made in society's attitudes toward fat people generally and fat women in particular.

On the other hand, thin women who are consumed by the need to get even thinner undoubtedly have an *internalized* problem, but they do not have to cope with the harassment and discrimination which many fat women encounter on a regular basis. Fat women must bear the additional burden of the external realities of weight prejudice, while thin women, for all their anxieties and fears, can still see their general body type celebrated throughout the culture. They do not have to go to special clothing departments, nor must they contend with the arrogance of some medical personnel who either blame any illness on weight or who humiliate and scold, neglect and mistreat, in the name of good health. They need not deal with the ubiquitous social ostracism which so many fat women suffer at one time or another in their lives. And while it's certainly true that some anorexics and bulimics were once heavy women who were driven to the wall because they could not bear to be laughed at and left out any longer, it's important to recognize that it was weight prejudice that originally backed them into that corner.

> *All through my school years, I wished I were dead rather than having to face another school day with people calling me "blimp," "chubby," "earthquake," etc.... One day I decided I would lose weight once and for all....Weight became my obsession, and I became anorexic, going without eating until my doctor—against my will —put me in the hospital and told me that in three more days I'd have dropped dead of a heart attack at 18....I'm 24 now and still struggling with anorexia.*
>
> Lisa Ames, "What it feels like to be fat," Minton
> *Parade* magazine, 1992

Working Towards Visibility

Is there a way out of this bad American dream? If so, it involves a more balanced and inclusive set of social standards. After all, given the increasing numbers of American women who wear a size 14 or over, it's neither reasonable nor logical to exclude them from the mainstream. Still, there is great resistance to the size-acceptance movement because it disturbs the closed-system, social status quo; it attempts to inject new and broader (so to speak) criteria into the stagnant thin-is-in pecking order. It also seeks to wean women off yo-yo dieting and thus threatens the weight-loss industry with a sizable redistribution of wealth.

The situation is not altogether hopeless, however. The fashion industry, which traditionally has not been the heavy woman's ally, is finally responding to her desire for attractive clothing and her ability to pay for it. As a result, ads for large-size clothing can occasionally be seen in the media, even though some retailers still insist on using thin models to advertise such products, thus demonstrating that they are quite willing to take the fat woman's money but would prefer to do so without publicly acknowledging her existence. Nevertheless, if large-size clothing maintains, even expands, its commercial niche—and there is no reason to assume that it will not—big women may yet live to see the day when they have equal floor space with smaller women and equal time in advertising, thus becoming regularly visible in at least one small aspect of daily life. True, it's a commercial, rather than a political, solution, but given the nature of American culture, that's an appreciable beginning. Big people who want to fight prejudice from within the system may find that the way to the mainstream culture's heart is ultimately through its corporate bottom line. Unfortunately, if the history of other rights movements has taught us anything by now, it's that even the most moderate social and political changes can take decades to effect.

In the meantime, fat people have an uphill battle on their hands. They must insist upon being judged as individuals rather than as a collection of measurements and body parts in a culture that pretends to appreciate depth and diversity but which is, in fact, philosophically conformist and materialistic. They must demand equality in a society which poses as classless but which actually relies upon a caste system based upon everything from race, gender, and age to shape, size, and physical ability, to determine who is or isn't considered deserving. They must raise their voices in a world that insists on seeing or hearing them only when it is convenient, and then only on its own narrow terms. It is a battle they cannot afford to lose.

> *What do we ask for? We ask for equal rights as American citizens. We ask for life, and the doctors to cure us, not kill us. We ask for equal access to public accommodations without fear of ridicule, and we ask for freedom of opportunity based on our potential, not our appearance. So let freedom ring.*
>
> Russell F. Williams
> "Let Freedom Ring"
> *The NAAFA Workbook*

CHAPTER TWO

The Health Police

Your Body Is My Business

I hate the impudence of a claim that in fifty minutes you can judge and classify a human being's predestined fitness in life....I hate the abuse of scientific method which it involves. I hate the sense of superiority which it creates, and the sense of inferiority which it imposes.
Walter Lippmann
In The Name of Eugenics
by Daniel J. Kevles

*O*n the subject of health, the invisible woman is caught fast between an irresistible force and an immovable object. Whichever way she turns, wherever she looks, she is judged and condemned as inherently unhealthy. Even if some people will concede that heaviness need not equal ugliness, there is a fixed determination that a fat woman is by definition a receptacle of disease. As a result, she can never do anything right unless she's losing weight. Eating a reasonably balanced diet, exercising regularly, not smoking, not abusing alcohol or other drugs, etc., is not enough. If she is not thin, she is not well.

Conversely, thin women are assumed to be healthy purely on the basis of appearance. Even if they smoke, drink excessively, abuse drugs, don't exercise, tan themselves into a precancerous state, suffer from eating disorders, practice unsafe sex, and so on, they are superficially judged to be fit in body and mind as long as the consequences of their actions are not visible. If a thin woman regularly consumes high-fat foods, the act is meaningless provided she remains thin; but let a fat woman do likewise, or express real pleasure in food, and she is seen as displaying a neurotic preoccupation or a dangerous disregard for her "unhealthy" size.

Heavy people, then, often find themselves at the mercy of the social phenomenon popularly known as the Health Police, that legion of fitness-preoccupied busybodies who see all of life from the perspective of numbers on a blood-pressure cuff or weight scale. Mr. Lippmann, just quoted, finds it "impudent" to "judge a human being's fitness in life" in fifty minutes, but the Health Police can easily beat that time: they'll do it in fifty seconds. By sheer virtue of their size, large women are forced into the ranks of the diseased, the disturbed, and the invisible.

Rationalizations and the "Health Argument" Hoax

This book will not argue about medical research and statistics concerning weight and health. I am not a doctor, and books such as *Fat Is Not A Four-Letter Word* by Charles Roy Schroeder, Ph.D. and *The Dieter's Dilemma,* by William Bennett, M.D. and Joel Gurin, together with others, have already accomplished that task far more effectively than I possibly could. Are there unhealthy fat people? Of course. But there are also many people who are unhealthy and thin and, more significantly, healthy and fat.

> *Being fat reflects neither weakness of character nor neurotic conflict; it is a biological fact of life, an aspect of the human species' inherent variability....The idea that health automatically benefits from weight loss is dubious at best. Nobody has ever proved that losing weight prolongs the life of moderately fat people, much less those of average weight. On the contrary, fatness itself appears not to be a major cause of disease, as we have been told it is.*
>
> Bennett and Gurin
> *The Dieter's Dilemma,* 1982

Flying in the face of such evidence, weight prejudice is predicated in large part on the false assumption that all big people are compulsive overeaters who are automatically sick and have willfully chosen to be that way, and also that this self-inflicted infirmity justifies all sorts of discrimination against them. The general public reads and hears *ad infinitum* that fat is a nutritional demon to be shunned, and extends that perception to include all fat people; eventually, the individual becomes invisible while only the fat is seen. This attitude assumes, in turn, that thin people are, relatively speaking, paragons of physical perfection, a stretch of the imagination so fantastic, yet so popular, that it could only be the product of an irrational cultural prejudice. Even when thin people do suffer from eating disorders, medical science uses special words— bulimic and anorexic—to distinguish them from healthy thin people; but there are no such special words for heavy people with eating disorders precisely because it is assumed that *every* large person is to some extent a physically inactive, dysfunctional overeater.

Still, if poor health habits alone truly justified the relentless harassment and discrimination that fat people often face, then many millions of thin people engaging in various compulsive/addictive forms of behavior would have to join the line to the woodshed, and a very long line it would be, too. Furthermore, if fat people attributed every case of thinness to anorexia or bulimia, much as the Health Police attribute every so-called extra pound to compulsive eating, the shouts of protest and accusations of prejudice would be deafening.

Indeed, experts and laypersons alike love to make a tremendous song and dance about the unwholesomeness of "excess" weight. In reality, the health issue is just a smokescreen. The zealots of the weight-loss brigade are fond of saying that "fatties"—a pet term meant to diminish and embarrass fat people—will grasp at any flimsy excuse to support their gluttony, but the truth is that it is weight bigots who will seize any lame alibi to justify their ill-treatment of big people, and the rationalization about fat being unhealthy is an all-time favorite.

In *The Nature of Prejudice,* Gordon Allport speaks of "defensive rationalizations," writing that "The most obvious way to buttress one's prejudices, and therefore to preserve them from conflict with ethical values, is to marshal 'evidence' in their favor" (1958). In other words, every time a weight bigot reads an article about the "dangers" of fat, she will wield those studies and statistics like a club to maintain her position of physical, even moral, superiority over all heavy people as a group. If she knows even one fat person with diabetes or heart disease, she will take it as incontrovertible proof that all fat people are likewise self-destructively diseased or destined to become so. If she sees even one fat person eating a large quantity of high-fat food, she will apply that perception to include all fat people. Conversely, the sight of a large woman exercising or eating dietetic food is typically greeted with a mixture of pity and contempt or a mental shrug to the effect that this woman is merely an exception to the rule. Either way, the large person cannot win.

Finally, the health argument represents what I like to call the "show me" trap into which many outsider groups are apt to fall; i.e., they are expected to prove time and again that they do not possess the negative qualities which are relentlessly attributed to them. Equal opportunity and simple decency are made contingent upon such proof. Thus, the African-American is continually made to feel the need to prove he/she is not a violent thug or a lazy welfare mother; the Jewish person is supposed to bend over backwards to display a lack of greed or pushiness; women feel obligated to don power suits and imitate men in the business world to show they are not weak and irrational; and large people feel a constant pressure to jump on the latest diet bandwagon and/or submit to questionable drugs or surgery to demonstrate that they are not heedless gluttons.

Ironically, although most commercial weight-loss methods are promoted as a simple and effective means of improving a woman's health, diets in fact typically trigger the yo-yo syndrome where weight lost is eventually regained together with additional pounds. This process is almost guaranteed to damage or destroy a big woman's health in the long run, hence creating a self-fulfilling prophecy. In any event, it is not just so-called extra pounds which the fat woman is trying to lose when she submits to a diet; she is also trying to escape the extra emotional weight dumped on her back in the form of social condemnation.

The Myth of The Slender Superwoman

Society is quick to malign large people based on their supposedly peculiar lack of good health, but are thin people truly the superior specimens they are supposed to be? Indeed, if thin America really takes health as seriously as it likes to pretend it does, then why is it still common enough to see smoking advertised as glamorous and sexy? People have known for decades that this is an unhealthy habit, and yet the public is still confronted with an endless array of ads featuring slender, chic men and women holding cigarettes and looking happily out at the audience, as if they were having the time of their lives. Also, many women smoke purely to reduce their appetites and keep their weight down, a practice which hardly reflects a concern for good health.

To the degree that women keep smoking because of their fears about weight, they are dying because of their fears about weight. (Krogh, 1991)

Likewise, humankind has for centuries been familiar with the ravages of excessive drinking; but again, liquor ads portray beautiful, thin people leading seemingly enchanted lives.

However, when food products are advertised—surely another "forbidden" pleasure if they are high-calorie, high-fat foods—one never sees smiling heavy people sitting down to a hot-fudge sundae or jumping about while eating a candy bar, even though they are presumed to be the primary, even the exclusive, consumers of such products. Apparently, big people are to advertisers of food—even diet food—what alcoholics and cancer-ridden smokers are to advertisers of liquor and cigarettes: an embarrassment to be kept out of sight. Needless to say, the manufacturers of high-fat or junk foods are perfectly happy to take the fat person's money; they just don't want to acknowledge her existence.

I recently decided to play my own version of one of society's favorite games: watching what other people eat. Having been the designated "watchee" in this pastime often enough, with anyone thinner being the "weight watcher," as it were, I thought it only fair to engage in a little discreet observation of slender women's eating habits, since they supposedly differ so dramatically from those of heavy people. The first thing I noticed during this exercise was that I had to make an effort to notice what thin women were eating. Why? Because militant though I may be on this subject, I failed to reckon with one of the more obscure rules of this game: the thin woman can eat anything she likes *because* she's thin; i.e., while big women who eat healthy diets are rarely acknowledged, thin women who gobble fattening foods are carefully overlooked, or at least excused. If the slender woman eats a hot-fudge sundae, that's all right because she "probably won't eat anything else all day;" if she has two slices of pepperoni pizza for lunch, that's okay because "she probably exercises a lot." Sitting in a restaurant one evening, I pointed out to my thinner dinner companion all the slender women around us consuming foods loaded with fat, to which she immediately replied, "Well, this may be the only fattening thing they eat all week." In similar situations, people might say, "Maybe she's buying it [the fattening food] for someone else," or "She probably won't eat it all." How do they know? They don't; they simply see whatever accommodates their stereotypes; and I found I had to shake myself mentally free of such assumptions for my little experiment.

What did I see? I saw thin women ordering super-sized burritos and nacho plates. I saw them eating ice cream, chocolate, cookies, cake, fruit cobbler a la mode, chips, pizza, doughnuts (big ones, crullers or custard-filled with chocolate frosting), gooey pastries, croissants smeared with butter or filled with ham and cheese, lasagna, candy bars, buttered popcorn, salami sandwiches, steak tacos, bagels smothered with cream cheese, and breakfast fast food. I overheard a very slender woman known for her candy habit tell her secretary that she was going out to get snacks, not because she hadn't eaten lunch but because she was "bored." I listened in on an elevator conversation between two thin women, one of whom was holding her stomach and saying, "I ate two plates!" I heard a man in my office teasing a thin woman carrying a box of Milk Duds, saying to her, "You're always eating candy." I watched as a slender co-worker ate junk food for breakfast and/or lunch day after day for weeks. So much, then, for the cliché of the slender person as a paragon of healthy, Spartan, "eat-to-live" food choices. So much, too, for the rationalization of weight prejudice based on a so-called concern for the fat person's health.

In a 1991 newspaper article examining health insurance discrimination against fat people, who sometimes are forced to pay higher premiums for health coverage (if they can get coverage at all), the director of the New York Business Group on Health was quoted as objecting, "Why should I pay extra premiums to pay for the health-care costs of other people with conditions that are readily preventable? Where is the equity?" (Privitere, 1991) Here is a statement just loaded with comfortable assumptions, the first of which is that being heavy is both a disease in and of itself and a condition that is easily altered. Just ask the majority of dieters who, after years of yo-yo dieting, are unable to keep off the weight for any length of time how "readily preventable" their situation is. Also, since medical science has at long last concluded that yo-yo dieting places a considerable strain on the heart (Haney, 1991), the idea that fat people should be coerced into yet another ride on the diet rollercoaster is counterproductive, to say the least.

Another sweeping generalization is that every heavy person eats large quantities of high-fat, high-cholesterol, unhealthy food. In fact, according to Drs. Rachael Heller and Richard Heller, authors of *The Carbohydrate Addict's Diet,*

> *For decades, researchers have tried to discover a link between overweight and overeating....The results of the studies are surprising. Some researchers have tried to make people of average or "normal" weight become overweight. They have failed—even when normal people were fed as many as 3,000 extra calories daily....In other studies, some overweight people were shown to be able to maintain their excess weight even when their food intake was severely restricted. Experiment after experiment has shown that overeating does not always result in overweight; nor is overweight always the result of overeating....the fact is that time and again the tests lead to the same surprising conclusion: Many people who overeat do not get fat and many people who are overweight do not overeat.* (1991, p. 18)

Yet, despite such conclusions, one still encounters blanket statements like "Overeating...is something all fat people do," or "Did you ever notice thin people in restaurants? They leave one-third of their food, not always, but often" (Bockar, 1980). Personally, I have eaten countless meals with "thin people" in restaurants, and it's been my experience that not only do they often eat all the food on their plates but they also frequently order more food than I do. Many are the times I've sat across the table in a restaurant from a thin person whose appetite far outstripped my own. And how can I forget the tall, slender, young saleswoman who told me that she would eat "cookies by the handful," never exercise, and remain thin nevertheless? Then there was the very thin female co-worker who, upon my asking how she could eat so much high-fat food without gaining weight, said that her doctor told her it was her metabolism— her size had nothing to do with her eating or exercise habits. But most people see only what fits their view of things, and what they want to see is fat women stuffing themselves with sweets and thin women picking at fruit and cottage cheese. The truth, however, is a bit more complicated.

There is an underlying idea that thin people do not incur excessive health-care costs. Are there no thin people with lifestyle-induced high blood pressure or high cholesterol? Are thin people immune to preventable—or at least treatable—long-term addictions to tobacco, alcohol or other drugs that result in a significant burden on the health-care system? Are thin people never responsible for "readily preventable" car accidents caused by drinking and driving? Are they invincible in the face of stress (which is avoidable, to a degree) that can contribute significantly to heart disease? How about hormone-driven sexual decisions, also "readily preventable," that can result in everything from herpes to unwanted pregnancies to AIDS? Talk about tragic. Talk about expensive! How about thin people who never exercise, who eat lots of junk food—who, in fact, are encouraged by cultural biases to delude themselves that thinness alone will save them from illness or an early death? Where is the equity, indeed? It is heavy people who should be asking that question, and loudly.

Perhaps one unconscious benefit that the thin world derives from equating fatness with disease is that doing so creates an illusion that if a person stays thin she will (a) rarely or never become ill, certainly not seriously ill, and (b) not die for a very long time.

Thus, fat people are left standing hopelessly in the manufactured shadow of perpetual sickness and early death. Playwright Susan Griffin once said, referring to prejudice, "Whoever is made into a scapegoat is connected to death" (Fox, 1992), a statement that applies quite well to fat women. "It's her fault she became ill/died," weight bigots can safely think. "What can you expect when someone doesn't take care of herself and lets herself go?" The fact that people sicken and die every day of many different causes, indeed, even the fact that they themselves must one day die, can be safely hidden away and ignored. Who's in denial now?

Ironically, many of the women who are the most obsessed with size, figure-watching, body-shaping, and exercise are thin or average-sized women. In her book *The Obsession: Reflections on the Tyranny of Slenderness,* author Kim Chernin describes her first episode of compulsive eating, which took place in Berlin. One minute she's enjoying a pleasant breakfast with some friends, and the next she finds herself running down the street stuffing rolls in her mouth, stealing a sausage from a German gentleman, frantically filling her mouth with the food, and tearing through bakeries and market stalls, buying more and more food, eating and running, eating and running (1981, pp. 4-7). This dramatic and harrowing passage may astound many heavy women who read it, not only because they themselves may never have experienced this kind of desperate compulsion, but also because they have been brainwashed to believe that thin women are all in perfect control of their lives and eating habits. Chernin's painful description of obsession only proves that it is high time our society gave up its cherished fantasy that body size alone is a reliable measure of physical and emotional well-being.

The reality is this: Research shows that fat people don't eat more than thin people. Research shows that fat people gain more if they eat excessively than do thin people (many of whom overeat with regularity). Research shows that when normally fat people and thin people undereat, fat people lose less. We have greatly overestimated the number of fat people who are actually overeating. But this research doesn't seem to discourage anyone from making judgments to the contrary. (Shaw/Wooley, 1991)

Exercise: Health Habits and Caste Systems

There is also the matter of exercise. According to statistics from the federal Centers for Disease Control and Prevention, only a small minority of American adults—between approximately 10 and 22 percent—maintain an optimal level of exercise (Roberts and Staver, 1992; Leary, 1993). Since fat people do not constitute 80 or 90 percent of the population, it's safe to assume that there are plenty of thin adults who can remain slender without exercising; yet it is big people in particular who are accused of couch-potato sloth. Exercise, like nutritious food choices, is seen as the magic wand that will make the fat person thin; if she merely feels great working out regularly, that's not enough—she has to *look* great by popular standards to be considered healthy. Fortunately, not all fat women have fallen for this line:

> *A great deal of my happiness and self-acceptance comes from being fit and healthy....I exercise regularly, both aerobically and using weight training, maintain a blood pressure of 110/60, and eat a vegetarian diet—eating anything I want. For a fifty-year-old woman, that ain't bad! My personal physician has confirmed my suspicion that I am in excellent health, so I am not just fooling myself.*
> Letter to *Radiance* magazine,
> 1991

Big women, like their thinner counterparts, typically face the usual obstacles to regular exercise: time constraints, jobs, commuting, demands by family and friends, and boredom. However, the fat woman has an extra hurdle to clear. The popular equation that fat equals pathology and thinness vitality also can contribute to a self-fulfilling prophecy for some heavy people, who are so accustomed to being told they're bad, ugly, and unhealthy that sooner or later many begin to believe it. What is the point, some may well reason, of exposing oneself to humiliation in front of all those arrogant, aerobicized physiques?

> *Many fat people have experienced being stared at and ridiculed by others while they exercise. This is especially true for exercise done on public streets...but it also applies to exercising at health clubs. Exercise instructors often make disparaging comments about fatness, in order to 'encourage' exercisers to keep at it....Since many exercise instructors outwardly exhibit disdain toward fatness and fat people, it is not likely that many fat people will feel motivated to attend exercise classes. People who exercise in the privacy of their own home, in order to avoid public scrutiny, may fear ridicule from members of their own families.*
>
> Parker, "The Role of Stigma-
> tization in Fat People's Avoidance
> of Physical Exercise," 1989

Not surprisingly, exercise illustrations in weight-loss books almost always use thin people to demonstrate the exercises, even when they are supposedly designed for heavy individuals. As always, the invisible woman is carefully kept out of sight while her thinner counterparts instruct her how to move, how to eat, and how to live.

Exercise is not always about health, anyway; sometimes it's about class and social status. Again, according to Jaclyn Parker:

> *Much of our society's preoccupation with slimness has more to do with attractiveness than health. A recent study by Hayes and Ross (1987) demonstrated that many people are motivated to engage in healthy behaviors out of their concern for their appearance; the authors suggest that the*

*recent trend toward exercise and physical fitness is partly
motivated by people's attempts to conform to a smaller
ideal body size, especially for women. They conclude that
when good health practices and appearance norms
coincide, women benefit;* **but if current fashion dictated
poor health practices, women might then engage in
those practices for the sake of attractiveness.** (1989,
p. 56; emphasis added)

Once, while scanning a local adult-education flyer, I found a listing for an exercise class which boasted that the class was
"guaranteed to leave you feeling self-righteous as well as looking
great." No mention was made of health-related benefits. Whoever
wrote this listing was obviously relying on snob appeal to attract an
audience; but any big person who's ever been on the receiving end of
this type of aerobic smugness knows how unpleasant it can be.

What Hayes and Ross fail to note in the preceeding passage, of
course, is that "current fashion" already dictates some abominable
health practices by intimidating millions of women into crash/yo-yo
diets, weight-loss surgery, diet-pill abuse, prolonged fasting, eating
disorders, compulsive exercise, and the like. We may never know
how much heart disease and other health problems can be traced to
destructive weight-control methods. The truth is, good health and
"good" looks are often mutually exclusive, a fact which tragically
carries no weight with millions of women who prefer conformity and
social acceptance to a private sense of well-being and a position at
the bottom of the social heap.

In Richard Simmons' book, *Never-Say-Diet,* he has what he calls
"The Very Painful But Very Honest Image Test" so that fat people can
measure their self-image. Simmons interprets a high score to mean
"[Y]ou are...delighted with yourself as a fat person and plan to enter
your own body in the Rose Bowl Parade next year as a float" (1980).
In dismissing walking as an inadequate exercise, he writes:

So you have a better heart after knocking your brains out and leaping over puddles and poodle stools. So what? Do you think when you walk into a room people say, "Hey, look at Helen's heart. Isn't it terrific-looking? Wow, I'd like to take her heart dancing some time soon." (p. 76)

Simmons' opinion is, not surprisingly, in direct contradiction with another hyperventilating weight-loss promoter, David A. Rives, author of *Walk Yourself Thin,* who claims that walking for an hour a day will give you the body of your dreams. According to Rives, "The worst day thin is better than the best day fat!" (1990) Self-satisfied, condescending remarks like these reveal a great deal more about the authors' priorities and self-images than about the people they profess to be helping. Of course, the Health Police are always ready to enjoy a giggle at the expense of a fat person's dignity. In fact, their livelihood often depends on it.

Obviously, health is not the primary goal here, but rather acceptance by others and rigid adherence to social standards. That imaginary thin person one hears so much about who's forever trying to climb out of a fat body is really a human being that the world just refuses to acknowledge unless she is properly cloaked in the minimum amount of flesh.

Prejudice for Profit

Indeed, many self-designated experts have a vested interest in maintaining the status quo of weight prejudice, since it provides them with such a convenient and reliable source of income. It's a rare woman in this country who doesn't own a single book or tape by some authority promising to share the secret that will make her thin and fulfilled. Americans have been persuaded that doctors and scientists are essentially impartial if not necessarily noble; unfortunately, one cannot always count on professional detachment.

I have always been repelled by fat women. I find them disgusting: their absurd sidewise waddle, their absence of body contour—breasts, laps, buttocks—everything I like to see in a woman obscured in an avalanche of flesh.
                                        Irvin Yalom, M.D.
                                        (Winokur, 1992)

Weight prejudice supports a greed which cloaks itself in a hypocritical concern for health, much as the racist philosophy of the "natural order of things" once supported the American slave trade. In order to keep the multi-billion-dollar weight-loss industry afloat, purveyors of diet products exploit and manipulate the insecurities of all women, but especially big women, assuring them that happiness is just around the corner if they will use their self-loathing as a springboard to move toward the land of the living, the land of the thin. Of course, if being large were to become culturally acceptable, these merchants of misery would go out of business and women could live their lives in the present instead of the near or distant future (and with a tidy sum remaining in their pockets).

Have you ever noticed that virtually every ad for a diet program or book uses the same old hook? First it acknowledges the common dieter's lament that "simply nothing works," and then it conveys a solemn promise that *this* plan is genuinely different and that it alone can unlock the mystery of permanent weight loss. Obviously, they can't *all* be the single miraculous answer to the "problem," or the hook itself would make no sense. Yet almost every product purports to be the long-awaited light at the end of the dieting tunnel, the one hope for success after all else has failed. And customers/victims keep coming back for more because they've been successfully persuaded that the penalty for failure is a lifetime of loneliness, sickness, and an early grave.

Moreover, a careful reading of many of the weight-control books of the past two decades reveals no small measure of twisted logic, self-hatred, and blatant bias. Advanced degrees or no, some members of the medical and psychiatric professions are more than happy to put their prejudices on display and make money at the same time. Do they ever take into consideration the growing body of evidence disputing the cause-and-effect relationship between fatness and illness? Do they ever believe a big woman who says she really isn't a glutton? Hardly. They are too busy literally making large bodies their business. In fact, the weight-loss industry relies heavily on the genetic/metabolic trap of cyclical weight loss/weight gain for repeat business. It capitalizes on weight prejudice while millions of people torture themselves with yet another last-chance, end-of-the-road diet.

Different weight-loss "experts" have long had all sorts of interesting ideas as to how to prevent or cure what they term obesity and its attendant problems. But neither a balanced diet nor good health is necessarily what's being sold. On the contrary, some diets, even those prescribed by M.D.s, are bound to cause more problems in the long run than they will cure. *Doctor Schiff's Miracle Weight-Loss Guide,* for instance, illustrates the dangers of accepting a doctor's word as gospel. In his 1974 book, Schiff promotes a maintenance diet that includes high-cholesterol items such as "roasts, chops, steaks, filets, racks, ribs, and rumps;...egg dishes and cheeses galore" while suggesting that "the limit is still one piece of fruit a day or one five-ounce glass of juice" (pp. 202-203). It isn't difficult to guess which are the doctor's favorite foods; but as a well-rounded nutritional plan, this one leaves a great deal to be desired. Going back a few decades, it's worth noting that Robert Cameron, author of the 1964 smash bestseller *The Drinking Man's Diet,* which promoted a diet of steak and red wine, probably no longer follows his own sage advice since undergoing a coronary bypass (Carroll, 1992).

The Last Chance Diet, promoted by osteopath Robert Linn in the late 1970's, was a liquid protein regimen that proved both popular and lucrative. It resulted in FDA documentation of "at least fifty-eight cases of people dying while on the Prolinn diet." Apparently, there was considerable risk to long-term users of "either sudden death or death due to intractable cardiac arrhythmias in individuals with no previous history of heart disease" (Mirkin/Foreman, 1983).

Joyce Bockar, M.D., in her 1980 book *The Last Best Diet Book,* heartily recommends what she herself describes as a "totally unbalanced...binge-and-starve" diet, an all-protein, ketosis-promoting regimen with "no vegetables, no fruits, no foods made with flour" (p. 197). According to Dr. Bockar, big people—she calls them "fat-persons," using the hyphenation to define them solely in those terms—are too set in their ways ever to change their uncontrolled habits, so they might as well be unhealthy and thin rather than unhealthy and fat.

> *Which way would you rather have it? A shorter life span, at worst (and damage from binging and starving has not been proven), but being thin, or a shorter life span from binging and being fat?* (p. 146)

Then there is Barbara Edelstein, M.D.'s *The Woman Doctor's Diet For Women,* a "national bestseller" published in 1977. This work attempts to separate itself from the pack by proposing that since the author is herself a woman, she is infinitely more knowledgeable about the female body and female needs than male physicians. Not only does Dr. Edelstein "occasionally use a short, intense crash diet for fun and variety" (p. 6), but she also sees nothing wrong with the use of thyroid hormone, although she admits that "the purists" (i.e., any doctors who disagree with her) consider such a procedure risky. Nor does she object to prescribing amphetamines (diet pills) for her patients because, according to her, big women are "much too fond of food...to become addicted (to the pills)" (p. 66).

This is questionable advice indeed, given that, according to the authors of *Over The Counter Pills That Don't Work,* even diet pills available without a prescription, like those containing PPA (phenylpropanolamine hydrochloride), a drug "originally marketed as a nasal decongestant" can cause "potentially fatal heart problems, kidney disease and muscle damage" as well as side effects such as "accelerated pulse rate, tremor, restlessness, agitation, anxiety, dizziness and hallucinations" (Kaufman, *et al.*, 1983).

Woman vs. Body: The Holy War Against Fat

In its relentless pressure to force women into a rigid mold, our diet-happy culture demands that a woman go to war with her own body. As most dieters have learned the hard way, the human body makes no allowances for hysterical cultural fashions; it often reacts to a restrictive food plan as a threat to its survival, trying valiantly to keep at least some of its "excess" fat, while women are sternly urged to dispose of it all as quickly as possible, by any means possible. The irony here, of course, is that fat women are consistently accused of ignoring their internal, biological hunger signals, supposedly overeating in response to external stimuli such as emotions or social events. How odd, then, that if a dieting woman employs these same methods in her weight-loss program—i.e., if she ignores internal, biological hunger signals like headaches, fatigue, hair loss, irritability and other symptoms of rapid weight loss as her body cries out for proper nourishment—she is hailed as a "winner" with a new and improved sense of self-esteem as well as a healthier body. If she "overeats" in response to taunts about her size, she's a neurotic failure with a poor self-image; but if she undereats, half-starving herself, in response to the same taunts, she's praised for displaying a healthy self-respect. What hypocrisy!

By now we're all familiar with the litany of doom laid down by the medical profession for anyone uninterested in starving herself in the name of thinness. Heart disease, high blood pressure, diabetes, gout, hirsutism (excess hair in women), increased risk of cancer, kidney problems, arthritis, etc.—how many times have we heard it? Given the austere authority and vehemence with which such pronouncements are usually made, a large woman might be forgiven for thinking it only a matter of time before she became a plague-ridden monstrosity rotting from the inside out. But where is the endless parade of articles about the illnesses incurred by drastic weight-loss measures? In fact, many of the adverse effects indicated by extreme dieting, fasting, drugs, and the like are interestingly similar to those supposedly caused by "excess" weight, although medical science seems to have overlooked this connection.

Fasting, for example, can cause arrhythmia and ketosis (a potentially dangerous condition resulting from fatty acids being released into the bloodstream) leading to acidosis "associated with gout" (Berland, 1974a). Regular use of appetite suppressants has been known to result in tachycardia (fast heartbeat), hypertension, ulcers, strokes, cardiovascular collapse, even death (Berland, 1974a, pp. 83-84; Schroeder, p. 137). Metabolism medicines such as thyroid, steroids, digitalis, human growth hormone (HGH), and diuretics may bring on complications ranging from decreased sexual desire to diabetes or a worsening of diabetes, rapid/irregular heartbeats, high blood pressure, and can also cause death (Berland, 1974a, p. 87; Schroeder, pp. 140-143). Weight-loss surgery (liposuction, stomach stapling, gastric balloons, etc.) has an extremely nasty laundry list of potential side-effects, only a few of which are irregular heartbeats, nerve and brain damage, impaired immunity, kidney stones, gallstones, anemia, fat embolism, stomach ulcers, stomach cancer, and death (Mirkin, 1983; Schroeder, pp. 159-160). Anorexia and bulimia can result in hirsutism, hypertension, cardiovascular problems, diabetes, kidney failure, and death (Squire, 1983, p. 224). And as for low-carbohydrate, ketogenic diets, it was known as long ago as 1968 that "in patients with cardiovascular disorders such as cerebrovascular and coronary artery disease, increased free fatty acids may induce cardiac arrhythmias" (Oliver, *et al.*, pp. 710-714).

A coincidence? If so, a most suspicious one. Medical science has miles to go before it discovers all there is to know about weight and metabolism, having only recently acknowledged, rather tentatively and half-heartedly, what most heavy women have had to learn the hard way: that diets don't work and in fact frequently serve to drive down body metabolism and foil weight-loss efforts. Yet for decades the pop-health practitioners of our time have arrogantly behaved as if every individual's weight and metabolism were matters as simply understood, and as simply altered, as a child's building-block structure or a piece of household plumbing.

Now, of course, the diet establishment can sit back comfortably and insist that it knows much more about nutrition and weight loss today than in the 1970's and 1980's. But how many big women conscientiously followed the diets described above, not to mention the thousands of others like them? How can anyone be sure that unbalanced and radical weight-control programs haven't caused or contributed to long-term damage infinitely more serious than hair loss and headaches, which Dr. Edelstein admits many of her patients suffer? If medical statisticians ever take diet-induced illness and weight gain into consideration when they spit out their countless studies about weight and health, they're keeping it a terrific secret. Even worse, consider this: if the diet-mongers didn't know everything "back then," what don't they know *now,* and how much more damage will they inflict upon people with their prejudice for profit?

The Invisible Killer: Stress

The emotional stress of being fat, in the United States, is not unlike that experienced by soldiers who spend long periods in a combat zone. Battle fatigue, of course, is more intense, but at least soldiers can be sent to rest and rehabilitation camps or sent home. Fat people in the modern western society are generally victims of excessive emotional stress during their entire lives. There is no relief even in solitude.

Charles Roy Schroeder, Ph.D.
Fat Is Not A Four-Letter Word

It's time to consider the question of stress as it relates to weight prejudice and so-called weight-related diseases. The annals of dieting are filled with hundreds of stories of fat women emotionally devastated by years of ridicule and humiliation, and yet their misery is ultimately attributed to their own failures as ignorant or uncommitted dieters rather than the failure of others to behave with simple human decency. On top of this is the smug insistence by many professionals and laypersons alike that even if a heavy woman isn't presently sick, she will be in the future. This outrageous assumption seeks to rob healthy fat people of the most basic sense of emotional well-being, as it demands that they live in dread of the future under a sentence of certain doom. Eating a reasonably balanced diet? It doesn't matter; lose weight. Exercising regularly? It doesn't count; lose weight. Don't smoke, drink, or abuse drugs? Don't engage in unsafe sex? That's not important; lose weight, or else.

Just being less heavy is never good enough for the Health Police. When I was a teenager, I managed to diet down to between 125 and 130 pounds, but my doctor had set a "goal weight" of 115 pounds; even now, I can remember the hunger headaches and fatigue as I exercised constantly, waiting desperately for that last plateau to give way (it never did). When I was in my twenties, I made it down to 140 and felt quite comfortable, but the counselor for the diet program I joined had set my "goal weight" at 125 pounds. For the doctor and the diet program, of course, this meant many profitable office visits and weigh-ins; but for me, it meant a perpetual state of tension and anxiety. All I knew back then was that I was sick of being laughed at and tired of always being on the outside of life trying to fight my way in; I had finally gotten a tantalizing taste of the social acceptance available to thin women, and I wanted more. So, I became yet another cog in that multi-billion-dollar wheel of fortune which is the American weight-loss establishment.

Do big women suffer from inordinate levels of stress? Just ask the woman who was disinherited and virtually disowned by her wealthy family for being fat. Ask the heavy teenage girl whose ever-critical grandmother told her that she waddled and it was no wonder she didn't have a boyfriend. Ask all the women who must endure being laughed at whenever they appear in public, or told pityingly that they have "such a pretty face," if systematic social disapproval isn't enough to wear out almost anyone. It cannot possibly benefit a woman's physical or emotional health to get the message that she ought to hate herself if she is large, and that other people have a natural right to pity, despise, or exploit her when it suits them. Nor can anything good come from reading supercilious self-help books whose authors insist that to be large is to be unfit in both body and mind, and that the big person will never be allowed to come in from the cold.

> You want a challenge? Take up bridge, or chess, or try to make some sense out of rugby. But don't keep challenging the world to accept you and love you as a fat person because it's never going to happen—no matter how many "fat-acceptance" groups spring up and no matter how many of them you join.

> Someone who is noticeably overweight has at least one more psychological problem than someone who isn't. Nothing wrong with that, except that "well" people don't want to be around "sick" people—psychological or otherwise. Not because they think the sickness will rub off on them, but because they know that, when the chips are down, such people are more likely to give in to their natural instincts and go running off into a corner somewhere with their cookies and milk, rather than digging in and toughing it out!

> They will never voice that concern—we humans are too nice to hurt someone else's feelings—but it will be the underlying reason why the fat person is never given jobs that he otherwise deserves, promotions that he's otherwise

earned, friendships that would be automatic if he were thin, etc....

If you want to have a better-than-even chance of being accepted, respected, loved, hired, promoted, etc., you're going to have to be thin.
David Rives
Walk Yourself Thin, 1990

How much stress, how much tension and illness are the result not of "excess weight" but of breathing such psychological poison day after week after month after year? How many sick hearts are broken hearts without hope, or hearts worn out by losing and gaining weight time and time again?

If I had a dollar for every hour I spent during my twenties and early thirties at home, watching television and crying into my popcorn because I was so lonely, I'd probably never have to work again. The social prejudice against fat people creates an environment where isolation for protection is understandable and all too common. Social prejudice is also a source of great stress, and the relationship between stress and the development of various illnesses has been extensively discussed in serious medical literature. What is not as well known is that people who experience life's stresses in isolation are at greater risk for both physical and mental health problems (Nuckolls, Cassell, & Kaplan, 1972). One could legitimately argue that the source of problems commonly associated with fatness is not the result primarily of weight, but is instead the result of lives spent painfully alone.
Lyons
"Fitness, Feminism and the
Health of Fat Women," 1989

Adding insult to injury, if the big woman does run into health problems after running a daily gauntlet of stress, it's quite likely that any such problems will be blamed on her weight. High blood pressure, for example, is firmly linked to high levels of stress, but she may be told to diet. If she gets an ulcer, she will probably be advised to cut down on rich or spicy foods. Having irregular heartbeats? Time to lose weight. Constant fatigue? Just drop those "extra" pounds, and everything will be all right. But is that really all there is to it?

In his book, *Why Don't Zebras Get Ulcers?*, Robert Sapolsky notes that, "finally, with enough stress, you become at added risk for developing adult-onset diabetes, one of the most common diseases of older people in Western societies" (1994). This is interesting, given that diabetes is one of the diseases so monotonously touted as being caused by "overweight." Even more interesting is Sapolsky's assertion that stress can disrupt reproductive processes, including female libido, another set of problems commonly attributed primarily to a heavy woman's weight. Most interesting of all is his statement that:

> *Some very careful studies are showing impressive links among stress, immune function, disease outcome, and longevity; in general, they have done a good job of controlling for age, health, socioeconomic status, smoking, alcohol consumption, physical activity, **obesity**, and use of preventive health services* (p. 151; italics added).

All this is certainly not to say that a fat woman is bound hand and foot to disease, but simply that if she does encounter health problems she should take into consideration her stress levels and any pressures placed on her by weight prejudice. It just may be that medical science has been putting the cart before the horse when it comes to big women and the so-called "weight-related" diseases. Indeed, in what has to be the height of irony, one recent Swedish study has reportedly linked stress to the development of abdominal fat ("Stress and Fat," 1993). In the end, society just might be forced to acknowledge that the burden pressing down so hard on the fat woman's heart comes not from the weight of her own body but rather from the crushing force of endless social criticism.

> *The harmful effects of chronic stress upon health and longevity is solidly established and alone could account for the statistical evidence that fat people die prematurely. Yet, stress has never been 'factored' into fatness research.*
> Schroeder
> *Fat Is Not A Four-Letter Word*

The Invisible Woman and Mental Health

Unfortunately, the boundless psychological damage done by weight prejudice is considered to be self-generated by fat women themselves rather than by the malice and ignorance of weight bigots. Much as women have in the past been collectively characterized as naturally overemotional and mentally chaotic, so, too, are large people specifically set apart as neurotic and self-hating.

> *Every time I see a fat person, I know that in some ways he or she wants to die; obesity is, after all, a slow form of suicide.*
> LeShan
> *Winning the Losing Battle,* 1979

Even while weight-control preachers readily acknowledge the ill-treatment of big people, they somehow manage to turn it around so that such behavior is always the fat person's fault. This skewed viewpoint results in statements like "Nobody loves a fat man (or woman, we add), especially not himself" (Rubin, 1972b). The list of emotional disorders commonly attributed, sometimes exclusively, to fat people, is long, oppressive, and sometimes contradictory. It includes: dishonesty (self-delusion); low self-esteem/self-hatred; envy—of all thin people, even, according to Dr. Bockar, "a whore or a pimp" (p. 34); compulsiveness; an unconscious association of food with parental love combined with an intentional use of "overeating" as rebellion against parental, spousal, or societal control; a fear of intimacy and sexuality; excessive anger; depression; a fear of rejection combined with antisocial tendencies; emotional dependency; laziness; pathological self-consciousness; and slovenliness.

Quite a catalogue, isn't it? Weight-loss writers often raise these spectres of mental disturbance to distinguish sharply between heavy and thin people, and are prone to smug and outrageous statements like, "Slender people usually don't hate themselves," and "A person with self-confidence and self-esteem is attracted to non-fattening foods" (Schiff, pp. 72, 73). One such book, *Psychological War On Fat* which, according to the back cover does "not admonish, preach, or prescribe," condescendingly refers to big people as "fatties" and contains an illustration of a heavy man as a human garbage can with an open mouth (Cordell, Giebler, 1977).

When young large women grow up reading and listening to hostile propaganda like this, it's no wonder that they develop a love-hate relationship with food and a variety of anxieties about their bodies. Not only can they expect to be condemned as physically unappealing and unhealthy for being even ten pounds over an "ideal" weight, but also as emotionally disordered. They quite rightly fear a bias so irrational and extreme that it describes them as even more degraded than the prostitute who must sell her body for money and the pimp who exploits her.

The Imaginary Shield: Fat as "Protection"

One of the many contradictions of weight-loss sophistry is the oft-heard cry that women are fat because they want to be, that they *fear* being thin, for somewhere in their disturbed minds thinness equals exposure and vulnerability. According to this rather bizarre theory, fat is not just "extra" weight but also serves as an additional boundary between a woman and society that not only keeps her safe from the world but also enables her to hide her true emotional problems from herself. According to David Rives in his book *Walk Yourself Thin,* if you become thin, "People will start giving you things to do that they would entrust only to people who are psychologically mature (which obese people definitely are not), so you'll have to start acting more like an adult" (1990, p. 63).

The question is, safe from *what?* From discrimination? Hardly. From the casual cruelty inflicted by weight bigots? No such luck. From loneliness and isolation? Not a chance. From responsibility? Some heavy people have no one but themselves to rely upon. The idea that fat people stay fat to protect themselves from "normal" relationships, success, and happiness relies upon the absurd premise that it is the fat person who has built a Berlin Wall of animosity and exclusiveness, rather than American society, which communicates quite powerfully its desire to keep big people at a comfortable distance.

In reality, it is thinness which actually provides women with a shield of armor behind which they may not be criticized. Society cloaks fat women in a shroud of mental illness while placing thin women on a pedestal supposedly built on a solid and unquestionable foundation of self-esteem. It is the large woman who is depicted as a wretched creature choked with conflict and self-hatred—*not* her thinner counterpart. It is the big woman who is consistently made to doubt her legitimacy as a female and a human being, *not* the slender woman. It is the fat woman who is typically presumed to be sick in body and mind regardless of her true habits, while the thin woman is held up as a model of pristine physical and mental health as long as the consequences of any bad habits or neuroses go unseen. If a woman wants to hide her personal problems, both from herself and the world, thinness is her best bet. As for the heavy woman, she is, as always, only visible as a misguided soul unconsciously regenerating her self-inflicted pain and perpetually in need of help from thin people—for a price, of course.

In the meantime, millions of American women continue to get caught up in eating disorders and ineffective, even dangerous, dieting techniques: starving, bingeing, vomiting, gaining, losing, worrying, sickening, even dying. The appetite-killing pills still sit placidly on the drugstore shelves. The diet books and diet programs keep coming, with their eager promises of self-fulfillment with self-reduction. The health articles continue to appear in newspapers and magazines everywhere, some saying one thing, others the opposite, each one claiming to have the final answer. Women may not learn much of substance about their health from all these dubious sources, but one thing they must learn if they are to reclaim their bodies from the specious diet peddlers and statisticians: that it is possible for total strangers to control a woman's body without ever laying a hand on it.

CHAPTER THREE

The Mass Media

One Picture is Worth a Thousand Diets

*Loyalty to petrified opinions never yet broke a chain or freed a human soul in **this** world—and never **will**.*
Mark Twain

*I*n our consumption-addled culture, the mass media encourage us to absorb as many goods as possible far beyond the saturation point. We are urged to buy things we don't really need and luxuries we may not be able to afford. Not only is more better, but we are advised that it will also make us sexier or more successful. But this rule has one notable exception: if a woman is perceived as having consumed too much food, she finds she has committed a social crime. By projecting the image of gluttony onto the large woman exclusively, our society can deny and rationalize its colossal overindulgence in the cult of conspicuous consumption. Greed, after all, is hardly restricted to a preoccupation with food.

In any case, no book of this sort would be complete without an examination of the mass media and its overwhelming contribution to weight prejudice. Movies, television, magazines, newspapers, and preachifying self-help books all reinforce and amplify the ignorant stereotypes about fat people that America holds so close and dear; taken together, they constitute a framework of "petrified opinions" which few dare to question. In *Man and His Symbols,* Marie-Louise von Franz points out that:

> *Attempts to influence public opinion by means of newspapers, radio, television, and advertising are based on two factors. On the one hand, they rely on sampling techniques that reveal the trend of "opinion" or "wants"— that is, of collective attitudes. On the other, they express the prejudices, projections, and unconscious complexes (mainly the power complex) of those who manipulate public opinion. But statistics do no justice to the individual.*
> (Von Franz, 1964)

I did my research. I watched the commercials. I studied the billboards, magazine articles and ads. I carefully noted the size of characters in dozens of movies and television shows. I cut out article after article until my apartment became a miniature paper warehouse. This went on for several months before I realized this research was a waste of energy. Time after time I typed into my computer, "Ad for Product Such-and-Such, featuring thin women only," "movie featuring thin women only" or "movie featuring fat woman as minor character/stupid/loser/sexless sidekick." Over and over I noted heavy, bald, short, old, and/or bespectacled male characters presented as normal, attractive human beings, while heavy female characters were typically presented as shrill, obnoxious, asexual, mean, and unappealing.

A survey of merely eleven mainstream magazines, including *Vogue, Redbook, Time, McCall's,* even *Audubon* and *Modern Maturity,* turned up an astounding 645 pictures of thin women as opposed to 11 of heavy women. Scrutinizing the local newspapers over a period of several weeks left me with a body count of 221 thin women as opposed to nine large women; newspaper advertising inserts added another 288 pictures of individual thin women and approximately a dozen heavy women (most of whom were pictured in a single store flyer for large-size clothing). An examination of almost 160 commercials—after that point, it was either stop or incinerate the TV set—contributed 120 ads featuring thin women exclusively, 27 ads depicting heavy males, mostly in a normal or positive light, and all of 12 heavy women, half of whom, interestingly, were either African-American, older, or both. Of ads including fat women, one offered an evil old cartoon witch, another pictured two big women dressed as opera-singer Valkyrie types, and a third depicted *Alice in Wonderland*'s mean-tempered Red Queen. A more recent series of commercials for Snapple soft drinks featured a fairly heavy woman who read complimentary letters from consumers of the product; however, in most of the commercials this woman is visible only from the shoulders up, while the rest of her body is hidden by a very high counter. Ultimately, the burden of proof in this respect was no more than a counting exercise.

Just a cursory sampling of the way physical size is characterized in the media goes something like this:

"Fat jerk!" (Comic strip)

"fat pig" (thin actress describing herself pregnant)

"sweaty, overweight tabloid reporter" (*Doonesbury* comic strip)

"naked walrus" (*Cathy* comic strip)

"blimplike" (news article about Chicago police)

"sicker and slower and fatter" (Arnold Schwarzenegger referring to the physical fitness of American children)

"pudgy sweets-lover" (newspaper editorial)

"pudgy nonentity" (description of singer Paula Abdul)

"Tubby," "Chicken Fat," "a fat, sloppy, yelling, screeching banshee," "depressed and overweight" (all descriptions of Elizabeth Taylor by others when she was heavy)

"major loser...short, bald and overweight" (description of a TV character)

"Fat with spongy flesh, small eyes, bad teeth, and mottled skin..." (description of a character in a novel)

"a woman so fat she destroys furniture...performs a long, simulated bowel movement" (description of a movie character)
"oil slicks in bags" (nutritionist Covert Bailey)
"chunky monkey" (description of a pregnant actress)
"guests revile one another as fat lying slimeballs" (description of TV dating show guests)

After drowning in an ocean of slender female figures everywhere I looked, it was easy to see how women are persuaded that thinness equals happiness and fulfillment. The women of the media are not only overwhelmingly small but also smiling, self-satisfied, exciting, dynamic, romantically involved, and generally having a splendid time. Whether an ad involves a new household cleaner, cosmetics or perfume, a low-fat, low-calorie food (especially that), a car, or a kitchen appliance, the message is that thin women never really have to be depressed or lonely. The pretty woman is entitled to have her life come out right in the end, and if it doesn't, it is a tragedy. This is sheer marketing fantasy—and yet, as a society, we buy it, we eat it up, we swallow it whole and ask for more.

Books

The majority of books written on the subject of weight, however radical or enlightened they purport to be, nevertheless focus almost exclusively on women and their supposedly self-created obstacles to happiness—their so-called neurotic needs, their denial, their miseries and failures. The average weight-related book gives little more than lip service to the notion that many of the problems fat women face are in fact generated by cultural prejudice. They preach about changing eating habits, of eliminating this craving or that thought pattern, but rarely of challenging society's discriminatory attitudes. Indeed, most books on this subject begin by condemning the pressures placed upon women to be slender but end by reinforcing those pressures when the discussion turns to the plight of the fat woman and what can be done to help her lose weight. Each and every diet book author, of course, presumes to know exactly how all large people think and feel, especially if the author has been fat.

In *Doctor Schiff's Miracle Weight-Loss Guide,* the author lists no fewer than 141 "excuses" why fat people refuse to get thin, including "What do you expect, perfection?" (apparently, yes), "It keeps getting harder to lose" (which, as we now know, is quite plausible), and, oddly enough, "I'm on a diet" (Schiff, pp. 38-40). This type of book is predicated on the ludicrous assumption that thin people are always thin because they take great care with what they eat. Therefore, remove the desire, adjust the emotions, the thinking goes, and any woman will lose weight.

On the other hand, in *Thin So Fast,* Michael Eades, M.D. admirably refrains from making moral judgments about large people, yet focuses primarily on case histories, including his own, of people who, when young, ate the way fat people are *presumed* to eat—that is, excessively—and only gained weight as they aged. One female patient indicated that "she had been 'skinny as a rail' while growing up, and that her favorite foods were ice cream, hamburgers, pizza, and doughnuts, all washed down with soft drinks. She had eaten these foods without restraint yet had never gained a pound" (Eades, 1989). Eades contends that "Very few people begin their weight problems as children," thus ignoring those whose weight has a significant genetic component and who may eat considerably less than their formerly-slender counterparts while still remaining heavy in the long run. Also, Eades' discussion of post-pubertal weight gain firmly establishes the link between a rapid metabolism and a naturally slender body size (despite a healthy appetite). However, big women know from bitter experience that should they even hint at a similar connection between a large body and a slow metabolism, they will probably be accused of "making excuses."

Another misguided assumption one often finds in weight-related books is that psychological and emotional difficulties are somehow exaggerated in heavy women. The reasoning here seems to be that because a woman is physically bigger than average, her problems must likewise be larger. For example, in his book *Forever Thin,* Theodore Rubin, M.D. provides the obligatory lip service to the effect that everyone is to some extent neurotic, has a foggy self-image, and struggles with conscious as well as unconscious conflicts; nevertheless, he continually makes the point that fat people have *more* of these problems (Rubin, 1970). Likewise, Marcia Millman, author of *Such A Pretty Face: Being Fat In America,* writes: "While there is a parent-child element in all sexual relationships, whether conscious or not, this dynamic plays a larger part in the lives of fat women, or at least is more obvious in their relationships with men" (1980, p. 158). Millman, who fills her book with one negative account after another of unhappy, self-hating fat women—many of whom were abused as children and undoubtedly would have been troubled regardless of their size—tries very hard to say something new, but ends by doing a slightly different dance around the same old cliches.

If men are sometimes attracted to heavy women because of unconscious associations with their mothers, could this theory not be applied with equal accuracy to men who insist on dating only small women, or are they miraculously exempt from unresolved Oedipal complexes? Judging by the number of requests in personal ads for small women with large breasts, this hardly seems likely. Is a so-called motherly figure the only physical feature that might trigger such connections in a man's mind? And while we're at it, why is it that a man who likes heavy women is assumed to have an active mother complex, but a woman who loves a big man is not popularly assumed to have a father complex? Furthermore, if a man has been raised by a loving mother who just happens to be large, and he naturally associates largeness with love and therefore seeks that quality in a prospective mate, is that pathological? Millions of people of all shapes and sizes seek mates who remind them of a parental figure, whether loving or abusive. What is pathological is the presumption that men who despise and automatically reject all large women simply have normal, healthy "preferences," but that any man who happens to appreciate big women must be as infantile and disturbed as the women he admires.

Does this mean that there is no such thing as a healthy attraction between a man and a large woman? One might succumb to that stereotype after reading the average weight-related book. If the authors of most such works know of any heavy women involved in secure, happy relationships, they pointedly exclude them from their discussions. Millman's book was published in 1980, and the magazine *BBW (Big Beautiful Woman)* began publication in 1979, complete with a letters-to-the-editor column which is typically filled with correspondence from fat women who insist they live happy, successful lives and are sick and tired of forever being labeled as miserable failures. Are all these women, together with their boyfriends, lovers, husbands, friends, and families, living a lie? Is each and every one of them suffering from delusions of grandeur? A more likely explanation is that our obsessed society is simply uncomfortable with men who will not submit to its strictures about whom they should or should not love and who are secure enough in their masculinity not to be intimidated by women who take up space.

Millman is correct when she says that much of the misery endured by big women in America results from prejudice, but she also ultimately reinforces that prejudice by relating one interview after another of women who present very disturbed and hopeless states of mind. There is little substantive variety in these women's experiences, and while the cover of the book purports to "break the long silence," Millman ultimately does nothing to challenge the stereotype of fat people as typically wretched.

Specifically, she writes that fat women "develop a belief in our potential greatness in order to console ourselves for not being loved or accepted, but eventually the preservation of the fantasy seems to take precedence over being loved in fact." She then urges big women to give up "the need to be extraordinary, special, unconditionally accepted" (Millman, 1980, p. 205). This is a sad old saw. Millman conveniently overlooks the fact that people of all sizes often build themselves up unconsciously in compensation for some deprivation or inadequacy, real or imagined. At one time or another, we all like to think of ourselves as "special" and "extraordinary." We all like to dream that sooner or later life will give us what we deserve. Yet Millman wants the reader to believe that this mindset is exaggerated in fat women. Also, Millman's theory clashes sharply with another weight-related book, *Winning The Losing Battle,* whose author absolutely insists that fat women are afraid of losing weight because they are actually terrified of *becoming* extraordinary, special people (LeShan, 1979). Damned if you do, damned if you don't.

Millman further makes the odd distinction that "While most people have a clearer self-image...the fat person is too self-conscious and too marginal to count on the accuracy of her interpretations" (p. 77). Again, she sets fat people apart from thin people. In the first place, it is not the heavy person's self-image that is usually in question in personal encounters, but rather the image projected by others *onto* her that is often unclear. The big woman must always wonder whether she is dealing with a prejudiced or non-prejudiced individual, especially if she is in a potential dating or romantic situation.

We live in a world where legions of people of all sizes, shapes, and colors construct and maintain deluded and muddy self-images. But perhaps the most revealing part of *Such A Pretty Face* comes at the end of the preface when the author, though "overweight" by only twenty pounds, defines herself as a person with a weight problem, rather than as a woman who just happens to be average or a little larger than average. When Millman refers to thin people as "normal," there is no irony in her use of that word. There should be.

Ultimately, even while they apply blanket pejorative terms like "overweight" or "weight/eating problems," weight-related books sternly promote the idea that weight loss will not make all of a woman's dreams come true. While disputing this cultural fantasy is certainly a worthwhile endeavor, what the literature fails to point out is that American culture invests enormous energy in pretending otherwise, often creating a self-fulfilling prophecy. Why *shouldn't* a woman believe that life will be better when she is thin, when this is exactly the carrot that society holds out to her as motivation? Why wouldn't a woman think that love, success, and lifelong happiness will be handed to her on a silver platter, when all around her are people who ignore or ridicule her when she's fat and express appreciation and admiration only when she loses weight? Society puts big women in a double bind by telling them that they are repulsive and comical, if even slightly large, and then lecturing them out of the other side of its collective mouth that weight loss won't solve their problems. In one sense, this is true, but only because it is *not* weight that is the source of the heavy woman's alienation, but weight *prejudice.*

Television and Movies

The most obvious pattern in television and movies, other than the predominant absence of large women, reflects the unsurprising fact that heavy men, although they suffer from the same general type of discrimination as heavy women, are not as severely censured for being large. Size in a man is often considered either a sign of physical power or a matter of no consequence. In a scene from the movie *Diner,* a large man eats plate after plate of sandwiches in a diner, apparently trying to set a personal record. The main characters, all male, are watching him in awe and cheering him on; no cracks are made about his size or his appetite. It is utterly impossible to imagine a big woman playing the same scene.

In even a cursory review of mass media presentations, one finds many more large men than women. Take, for example, actors John

Goodman, the late John Candy (whose death has been attributed not purely to his weight but also to a rapid and substantial weight loss), *Cheers'* George Wendt, Bob Hoskins, the late John Belushi (dead of an overdose of drugs, not food), the late comic Sam Kinison (car accident, not clogged arteries), French actor Gerard Depardieu, and British comic Robbie Coltrane, to name a few. All these men have played characters who, although heavy, are nonetheless portrayed as lovable and appealing enough to attract thin, conventionally-attractive women. Can anyone imagine a female version of *Cheers'* Norm—a lazy, work-phobic, beer-guzzling woman who assiduously avoids home and husband—being hailed as funny, let alone "beloved," as one news article put it?

Goodman, although sometimes cast in negative roles such as a drunken slob (*Stella*), a corrupt cop (*The Big Easy*), and a moronic criminal (*Raising Arizona*), was nevertheless named in a 1994 *TV Guide* article as one of several "unlikely heartthrobs" which pronounced that "[s]ometimes concerned and cuddly beats buns of steel" (Mitchard, 1994); and television actor Dennis Franz, who is both balding and big, has been called "a sex symbol in the making" by the same publication (Rensin, 1994). John Candy was invariably paired romantically with thin women in his movies. Likewise John Goodman in *Punchline,* and Jackie Gleason in *The Honeymooners* and even in his old age, in the movie *Nothing In Common*. Ditto Bob Hoskins in his films (*Mermaids, Mona Lisa, Who Killed Roger Rabbit?*), and John Belushi and Sam Kinison in real life.

Of course, we're all well acquainted with that popular movie plot involving the sweet but physically unexceptional male who yearns after the beautiful, thin heroine and eventually, by means of his irresistible personality, wins his true love (*Minnie and Moskowitz* comes immediately to mind). In the film *Green Card,* a beautiful, thin woman marries a not-so-lovely Frenchman so he can emigrate to the United States, and although at one point she shouts at him, "You're a slob! You're overweight! You're disgusting!", she is nonetheless passionately in love with him by the end of the film. The male-dominated film industry never misses an opportunity to remind us that men should always be loved for themselves. But what about women?

When Hollywood was casting for the 1991 film *Frankie and Johnnie,* a story about an ordinary-looking woman who falls in love with a plain-looking man, Kathy Bates, an Oscar-winning actress who portrayed Frankie on the stage and who just happens to be large, was passed over for the film role. The part went instead to Michelle Pfeiffer, a thin, conventionally glamorous blonde who obviously wanted to prove that she could play a character role. This is typical. If the heavy woman has any consistent role in commercial American films, it is as the peripheral, asexual mother or "buddy," and rarely, if ever, the central, romantic character. Message to all large women: You're not sexy. The only beautiful woman is a thin woman.

Incidentally, some other roles Ms. Bates has been given in movies include an unhappy, divorced mother in the film *Used People,* a controlling and ultimately insane missionary in *At Play In The Fields Of The Lord,* an unhappy housewife in *Fried Green Tomatoes,* another unhappy housewife in *The Curse of the Starving Class,* a "widowed mother of six" in *A Home of Our Own,* and a violent psychopath in *Misery.* Bates herself pointed out in a 1991 interview that when she read for a part in the Sylvester Stallone movie *Paradise Alley,* the character breakdown showed that "after every single female character's name was the adjective 'beautiful,' even if the character was age 82." When Bates questioned the casting director about this, he replied, "Well if you want to make your own female version of *Marty* (a movie about a lonely, aging, unattractive man), be my guest" (Finke, 1991). A New York critic also made an offensive remark about her weight in a review of her stage performance in "Frankie and Johnnie." In other words, Bates is an extremely talented actress who has difficulty getting the parts she deserves solely because of her weight.

The double standard is also alive and well on television. On the *Soaps* page of a 1991 issue of *TV Guide* (Logan, 1991), one finds actor

Jerry Adler—described as a "Rodney Dangerfield lookalike"—flanked on each side by a thin, conventionally-gorgeous woman; one is smooching him on the cheek and the other has one hand on his chest. Picture the reverse, if you will: an old, thin-haired, chunky woman surrounded by two young male model types, one of whom is kissing her on the cheek and the other one with his hand on her breast. Will we ever see such an image in our lifetimes? Don't hold your breath. On one episode of the popular show *Cheers,* a thin, conventionally-attractive woman is shown pursuing a heavy, bald, bespectacled man romantically because she is what he terms a "chubby chaser." Wouldn't it be nice, once in a while, to see a gorgeous hunk pursuing a heavy woman with glasses? "Fat" chance!

On the other hand, one gossip-column item about large-sized comedienne Roseanne and her former husband, Tom Arnold, also a large person, at a public function described Mr. Arnold as wearing "black tie. She wore black tent!" (Smith, 1991) Although indisputably talented, Roseanne has had to endure endless vitriolic attacks based on her weight, such as when New York *Observer* columnist Michael Thomas compared her to the *Star Wars* blob monster, Jabba the Hutt (1994). When large actress Delta Burke was profiled in a national magazine, the front cover pictured her with an American flag draped before her, effectively covering up most of her body. When *TV Guide* interviewed her, the article was accompanied by pictures showing her only from the bustline up. Meanwhile, a "Grapevine" item in another issue of the same magazine presents a full-length shot of the somewhat hefty actor Peter DeLuise, stomach spilling over his belt and all, together with a blurb about his audition for *Studs,* a steamy television dating show (1992, p. 4).

Remarks made in front of the cameras are often no less offensive than those made behind them. In one movie, *Violets Are Blue,* a thin wife tells her husband, only half-jokingly, that she hopes his ex-girlfriend turns out to be "short, fat and ugly." In the 1984 film *Irreconcilable Differences,* Shelly Long's character overeats and gains weight after a divorce, and in one scene in a supermarket she glances at several heavy women who are, not surprisingly, all dressed in dowdy, cheap clothes. Horrified, she realizes she's turning into one of "them." In *City Slickers,* of the three male protagonists, two have slender, pretty, "good" wives. The third has a heavier, less pretty wife, who is, of course, domineering and unlikable. In *Steel Magnolias,* two thinner women sneer at a big woman who's dancing by comparing her hips to "two pigs fighting under a blanket." And in the film *Welcome Home, Roxy Carmichael,* one woman says to another of the title character, "I just can't wait to see if [she]'s been able to keep her weight down." In a scene from *The Golden Child,* Eddie Murphy's character encounters a man at a newsstand who is reading a porno magazine called "Chunky Asses." There is a picture of a large woman on the cover. After Murphy's character has embarrassed him, the man hastily puts the magazine back and walks away. Murphy then looks at the magazine and says, in utter disbelief, "Chunky Asses???" Sometimes just the sight of a big woman is enough to evoke a snickering mirth, as in *Shoot The Moon,* when four thin little girls see a big woman's face on TV and burst into derisive giggles.

Of the approximately 70 movies I randomly surveyed—mostly mainstream commercial American films—only 17 had any large female characters at all in the script, most of whom represented the standard domineering mother figure, the comically unattractive woman, the whore figure, and Bates as her *Misery* psychopath character. Only six of these 17 films presented a big woman as a positive figure, and of these six, only three—*Daddy's Dyin'—Who's Got The Will?* and John Waters' *Hairspray* and *Crybaby*—featured fat women as romantic figures and central characters.

Usually, though, a big woman is an anti-sex symbol. In a scene from the film *Reversal of Fortune,* a group of lawyers and law students discuss the circumstances of a case concerning a man and two women. All the female law students are, of course, thin, young, and attractive. While talking about one woman involved in the case who is "a 300-pound hooker with red hair and white boots," one of the women makes a sound expressive of disgust, and another one says, "He had a beautiful mistress and he went with an ugly whore?" One heavyset male student, speaking of the mistress, says, "...he was still in love with her. And why not? She's a babe."

Television shows are not much better, although they occasionally make an effort. Ricki Lake, who has since lost weight, was featured in the defunct series *China Beach,* Delta Burke once co-starred in *Designing Women* and had her own series; and Roseanne's show has long resided among the Top 10 in the Nielsen ratings. Although these women are encouraging examples of talent overcoming prejudice, they are too few and far between. At best, TV shows typically treat large female characters as special cases whose weight is always a matter of comment, rather than integrating women of all sizes and shapes into their programs as a matter of course.

One episode of an early 90's show called *Herman's Head* revolved around a woman from the title character's past who was once heavy but had since lost weight. Upon seeing a picture of the ex-classmate at her former weight, one of the voices in Herman's head called Lust—played, incidentally, by a heavy man—says, "Whoa! Is that just one woman?" Another voice, called Sensitivity, played by a thin woman, says, "Come on. She's just a little overweight. Besides, maybe she's lost some of it." Lust replies, "Great, now she's down to enormous!" But when they discover that the ex-classmate has lost weight, she immediately becomes a desirable sexual prospect.

On *L.A. Law,* heavy actress Conchata Ferrell played a new character who was dumped from the program after a relatively short tenure. Her role, that of a tough attorney, was variously described in reviews and on the show as "loud, brash and overbearing," "tubby," "aggressive," "bullying, overpowering," and "a real cash cow." At one point in the series, Ferrell's character marries a handsome, slender man amidst tittering speculation by the firm's slender female attorneys as to the groom's ulterior motive. Naturally, it turns out that he is a foreigner who has married the fat attorney solely to gain citizenship.

On an episode of *Married With Children* (which insults everybody and everything with no discrimination), a game-show contest involves squashing a man lying under a mattress by having fat women sit on it. The man's wife says, "Start the herd!" It is worth noting that no fat men were used in this particular scene, only women. And so as not to ignore cable programs, on an episode of HBO's *Dream On,* the main character has a dream in which he tells his secretary, a heavy woman, that he loves her "as a woman," and then kisses and embraces her. He wakes up screaming in horror from the nightmare. The woman's character is, not surprisingly, drawn as abrasive, loud, and pushy.

In a Disney cartoon about teenagers that apparently refers to the 50's or early 60's, a teenage girl is drawn by the cartoonist with large hips, and a nearby teenage boy yawns with obvious distaste. The girl looks indignantly at the cartoonist, who hastily redraws and reduces her rump to a smaller size; the boy immediately responds, grabs the girl, and they dance happily away. The problem, then, is not so much that, in TV and movies, bad women are always fat, but rather that fat women are so often deliberately created as unappealing characters.

Finally, another profitable but prejudiced assumption reflected in the mass media is that a robust appetite for food is solely a male prerogative. When a man eats, even a heavy man, it's seen as an expression of his gusto for life, his masculine appetites. One TV ad for cheddar cheese featured a heavyset man eating from a big plate of nachos, while a radio ad for a local supermarket chain had a chirpy woman talking about how every meal is a contest between her two sons and her husband as to who can eat the most. An ad for Pepto-Bismol pictured a man rubbing his rather prominent gut prior to using the product. Can you imagine ever seeing a woman doing likewise, or listening to a father brag about how much food his wife and daughters can eat? Then there's Swanson *Hungry Man* frozen dinners, featuring 50% more meat and extra portions, a product endorsed by Bubba Paris, a big football player. The implication, obviously, is that this is a food item for men. Can we look forward to a food product called Hungry Woman with extra portions? Don't bet on it. There's also Sloppy Joe *Man*wich, which advertises that it's "not just a sandwich, it's a real meal." And let us not forget the quite popular series of Round Table Pizza ads featuring a heavy man making and eating the product.

Not surprisingly, other than the Snapple commercials mentioned earlier, I could not find one example of a heavy woman endorsing food items. Scanning ad after ad for junk food, fast food, diet food, candy, cheesecake, condiments, beer, cereal, etc., they all featured—you guessed it—thin women leaping about, smirking, sipping, chewing, eating. The manufacturers of these products, of course, want as many people as possible to buy their wares, but since fatness is considered a fate worse than death for American women, fat women cannot be used to promote foods lest thin women associate their consumption with weight gain. If the invisible woman eats, then she must not be seen.

The Personals: "No Fat Women, Please"

How do I measure thee? Let me count the ways. Single/Divorced/ Married, White/Asian/Black/Hispanic, Christian/Jewish male seeks thin, slender, svelte, sleek, petite, willowy, lean, lithe, slim, trim, fit, athletic, weight-proportionate, not obese, in-shape, unfat, X-number-of-pounds female. An exaggeration? Not really. Although it's true the personals are not strictly part of the media establishment, they do constitute a public forum and mass-communication network, and they illustrate in a very raw fashion the reflection of media imagery in the desires of men.

The patterns of the personals reflect the usual stale stereotypes and sexism of weight prejudice. Out of 324 ads by men seeking

women in which the men specified body size, 312 requested, or
rather demanded, a thin body type—and employing, incidentally, all
the synonyms for "thin" listed above. Men have a most creative
vocabulary when it comes to describing a woman's body. Indeed, to
judge by the phrasing of the ads, "slender" and "attractive" are one
word, not two, in the same fashion as "fat" and "ugly." Some other
charming phrases also aptly express the touching importance of size
to many gentlemen advertising for their "soulmates:"

"Seeking attractive, thin woman, 100-120 lb. Your friends
jealously call you skinny."

"SWM, 40, 165 lbs.... seeks healthy lady, 95 lbs."

"Disgustingly wealthy J/M.... *socially conscious,* seeks tall,
beautiful woman, similar background. No fatties, golddiggers or
codependents." (Emphasis added.)

"Must look good in and enjoy wearing tank top/halter and shorts,
bikini, etc."

"WM, 5'10", 230 lbs.... prefer short, slim woman"

"5'9"...bald, wear glasses, need to lose 15 pounds... seeking...
slender to medium woman, not fat"

"Please be... height and weight proportional... I dislike people
hung up on... beauty."

Other men were also very clear about their requirements:

"Unfat, unshaven, latent nympho,"

"36-24-36,"

"somewhat fragile... very easy on the eyes,"

"busty a plus. No heavies,"

"Rubenesque won't work,"

"spankings... for petite women only,"

"you're not fat," "130 lbs. max.,"

"size 5 to 7,"

"95-135 lbs.,"

"good looks (7+),"

"100-125 lbs.,"

"non-porky." And so on.

It is most interesting that male admirers of big women are commonly portrayed as little boys looking for a mother figure; yet here, one finds men who appear to be looking for a very small, dependent, child-woman/daughter figure and status symbol. Could it be that they have their own peculiar incest fantasies? Not surprisingly, although women advertising for men often mention height as a requirement, they do not, unlike men, usually specify size and shape of discrete body parts. Thus, although one often sees ads from men seeking large-breasted or long-legged or long-haired women, one does not typically see ads from women demanding a particular penis length or waist size. Also, since men generally perceive size as power, it seems reasonable to consider that men with rigid, inflexible standards seeking very slim women much smaller than themselves may be looking for mates who not only provide them with social prestige, but who are easily dominated on a physical and possibly psychological level. Might one go even further and speculate that the preference for women with androgynous or boyish figures represents a closeted homosexuality in some men, or an unconscious fear of and hostility toward the more powerful femininity of the large woman?

It is also interesting to note that a great number of these men describe themselves as athletic types who enjoy working out. If most of them are being truthful, this suggests that at least some of these men spend the bulk of their spare time and energy maintaining their bodies, a relatively narcissistic pursuit, rather than participating in social and romantic relationships. Perhaps a woman's body is of primary importance to this type of man because he is so consumed with his own physique, and he wants someone who reflects his self-absorption. Unfortunately, in today's culture, this personal scenario passes for supreme, macho self-esteem—in a man or a woman. Like the slender, body-obsessed woman, such a man may have neglected his emotional and intellectual development and have little more to offer a woman besides money and muscles, so in fact he really is seeking his soulmate when he stresses the necessity of thinness and beauty above all else. One personals advertiser, having described himself, requested a "lady clone slim," and one wonders if a mirror wouldn't serve him just as well.

In any case, the overall impression of the personals is that men still care more about a woman's body and looks than her qualities as a human being. An S/B/M (single black male) summed it up perfectly when he wrote, in search of a woman who "weighs no more than 140. Be any race, be yourself, but be beautiful." Or else?

Newspapers

The problem with mainstream newspaper journalism is twofold: first, its hearty participation in the national pastime of describing fat people in contemptuous terms; and second, that it purports to be an objective, unbiased observer and reporter of news and culture. But when entertainment journalists describe a large actress as "a blimp on the way to full zeppelin status" (Miller, 1992) or a bone-thin actress as "delicately gorgeous," the reader can make a pretty good guess as to their personal views as well as their degree of impartiality.

Comic strips such as "Beetle Bailey," "B.C.," and "The Wizard of Id" routinely portray fat people, and especially women, as coarse, obnoxious, domineering types. Other strips, most notably "Cathy," feature female characters who know quite well that weight obsession is oppressive but nonetheless serve as its obsequious slaves. In editorials and other features, phrases such as "She's a blimp but she doesn't look bad" and "pudgy sweets-lover," headlines blaring "Americans Still Kind of Porky," and insulting comparisons—one newsmagazine contributor likened a herd of elephant seals to "a Weight Watchers' group in spandex"—reflect the same rancid stereotypes displayed elsewhere.

The language and images of the print media, like those of film and television, reflect a blind allegiance to weight prejudice. Here one finds full-figured women being advised every summer in the fashion column to wear silhouettes that act as camouflage and are "forgiving" to their flawed bodies, as if they had committed sins that required absolution. Another fashion article about designer stockings smugly advises that "on the large-limbed and lard-legged" such luxurious accessories "are no more than sausage casings," although "on good gams the look is luscious and the feel is exquisite" (Shapiro, 1992). An editorial about truth in advertising as to food fat content discusses the subject only as it relates to fat people, as if they were the exclusive consumers of high-fat foods. A health and fitness article about weight is accompanied by a drawing of a fat man in a bathing suit but with a pig's head and hooves. An editorial cartoon depicts a large and obnoxious husband and wife, flesh spilling out of their tacky, skimpy clothes, complaining indignantly to a newsdealer about the morality of actress Demi Moore's naked pregnant cover shot for *Vanity Fair* magazine ("This shocking public display of flesh oughta' be banned," Wilkinson, 1991). The message here is twofold: first, that the cartoonist personally classifies fat people as innately loud, boorish, and ignorant, and assumes that the reader will make the same association; and second, that it is the fat couple's overflowing flesh which constitutes the real affront to cultural sensibilities.

One of the best—or worst—examples of journalistic weight prejudice was the local sports columnist reporting from the 1992 Barcelona Olympics on the Spanish beaches, and his disparaging remarks about local older women possessed of the sheer tasteless gall to walk on said beaches in "nothing but" their swimsuits. This same columnist also deplored women who dared to sunbathe undraped on a topless beach—not because they were naked, but because they lacked the flawless breasts and figures that appeal so to the male eye (Nevius, 1992). It seems that not only must women limit their food intake to please men, but they are also expected to restrict carefully their style of dress and their activities, lest they distress delicate male sensibilities with exposure to "imperfect" bodies.

Even in newspaper articles that have nothing to do with diet and weight, women are frequently described in terms of their approximate or specific weight and appearance. Phrases like "tall sexy...type", "the mountain of blond hair she balances on 102 pounds," "slender beauty," and "California girl beauty" appear in one article alone about female stand-up comics which includes, interestingly, a graphic description of a man helping himself to generous portions of a buffet while the women sit and drink only water (Kahn, 1991c). One newspaper item about singer Ann Peebles refers to her as "the 99-pound vocalist" (Selvin, 1992); another article briefly profiling four blues musicians describes the one woman in the group as "5-foot-3 and 105 pounds" but makes no mention of any of the three men's physical attributes (Orr, 1992). In a *Parade* item about British actress Jean Marsh, the author points out that "even in her mid-50s (she) still sports a 19-inch waistline" (Brady, 1992). One wonders if this information comes with publicity kits or whether reporters simply bring tape measures and weight scales along when they interview women. Other articles, like the one about the late Audrey Hepburn gushing about her perpetually slender figure, or another about Elizabeth Taylor that babbles endlessly about her weight fluctuations, also focus unabashedly on a woman's body.

On the other hand, most newspaper items omit such detailed descriptions of men's sizes and body parts. One interview of director Robert Altman describes him in terms of his age and hair color, and compares him to a "bemused, slightly grumpy, extremely shrewd owl," but makes no mention of his weight, although the full-body shot accompanying the article reveals a clearly heavyset man (Guthmann, 1992a). An article in *Parade* magazine about the late large actor John Candy refers in the briefest and most casual manner to his 300-pound girth but never insinuates that he has a weight "problem," and the accompanying waist-up photograph of Candy obviously makes no apologies for his size. "Bearlike" seems to be a favorite adjective of journalists when describing heavy men. Perhaps most significant of all is the constant barrage of newspaper and magazine articles concerning female models—their trials and tribulations, their multi-million-dollar contracts, their glamour and dazzling beauty—and the virtual absence of similar articles regarding young teenage *boys* being set on the path to fame and fortune via modeling careers. Could it possibly be that, while model-style looks are still considered the pinnacle of success and the proof of social/sexual validation for a woman, they are not required to be a "real" man?

As for print advertisements, they lack the dynamics of television ads, and consequently they can come on quite strong in their promotion of thinness as the ultimate aphrodisiac. One diet product ad out of *TV Guide* depicts a thin woman in a leotard examining her hips. Superimposed upon the picture are the words "We'll help you turn on more than your metabolism." Next to the picture, the ad begins, "You're not only dieting for yourself. That's why it's so important to lose those extra pounds...." Another item in a different issue of this magazine hawks an exercise machine, and while the words describing the health benefits are in rather small print, the impossibly slender and leggy female model in the ad is quite noticeable, as are the words, "Hurry! Get that NordicTrack figure you always wanted." Then there are the ubiquitous exercise club advertisements featuring women who are dressed, shaped, and posed more like centerfolds than athletes or average people.

The mass media do not really reflect an idealized reality, as its gurus would like us to think. From the movie studios and directors, to the ad executives and the TV producers and the novelists, rock stars, and music video producers, the media masters have constructed a universe of "petrified opinions" where the only valuable woman is a thin woman, while big women function primarily as shrewish, silly, asexual mommy figures or cheap jokes. Not only is this one-dimensional viewpoint warped and oppressive, it is crashingly dull, redundant, and predictable. Taken as a whole, this so-called creative product conspires to turn impressionable young women into insecure nervous wrecks trying to compete with image upon image of the same tiny-waisted, big-breasted dream girl.

If art really is a reflection of life, and the mass media in turn are a businesslike imitation of art, then when Americans struggle and strive to shape their lives in the media's image, they are living life twice removed. The constricted vision of the world fabricated by Hollywood and Madison Avenue compresses the individual and her hopes, needs, and dreams into narrow channels, reducing life to a hopeless pursuit of false perfection in imitation of people who exist primarily for the illusions they can project. And what *Boston Globe* columnist Ellen Goodman has written about women's magazines can be applied just as easily to the entire media machine:

> *Flip through* **Elle, Allure, Mirabella, Harper's Bazaar, Glamour, Mademoiselle, Vogue,** *and you see messages on a collision course. The magazines are both critiquing and promoting the beauty industry. Critiquing the images of flawless, lineless, hipless beauty and promoting flawless, lineless, hipless cover girls. There are thoughtful essays about the dangers of anorexia alongside photographs of models, role models, who are anorexic waifs....The message is that you can be brainy even if you're beautiful and that you'd better be beautiful even if you're brainy. There is, literally, no money to be made in telling women to feel good about themselves* ("Beauty Queens And Platforms," 1993).

"Be any race, be yourself, but be beautiful." Or else.

CHAPTER FOUR

Weight Prejudice and Sexism

The Invisible Woman as Failed Sex Object

Food is the primal symbol of social worth. Whom a society values, it feeds well. The piled plate, the choicest cut, say: We think you're worth this much of the tribe's resources.
Naomi Wolf
The Beauty Myth

I think you may have to have a tiny touch of anorexia nervosa to maintain an ideal weight...not a heavy *case, just a little one!....Can you admire your utterly outstanding pelvic bones the way other people admire Bo Derek's bosom, take endless pleasure in patting your stomach because it (still) isn't there, thank God!, go into* deep *depression at the gain of even* half *a pound? Good!*
Helen Gurley Brown
Having It All

*M*ost of us are familiar with the fact that large women were at one time considered extremely attractive. Painters such as Rubens and Renoir portrayed the voluptuous female figure as the essence of beauty and vibrant life. It's also a fact that from the dawn of humanity a large woman has symbolized fertility, nourishment, and survival. What does all this mean to us now? Large breasts are certainly still in style, but what about the rest of the female body? Why is a boyish figure in a woman glorified and a more robust form vilified? It seems painfully obvious that the modern American attitude toward female flesh—an attitude, it must be said, that is not shared by all other cultures—reflects a deep-seated hostility toward femininity in its most primal, organic shape. Nor does this hostility stop at the surface, since, as we have seen, a host of negative qualities is consistently attributed to the heavy woman.

It does not go too far, I think, to say that this irrational attitude toward large women mirrors an unconscious collective male attitude toward femininity as a concept and women as a group. This is why the predominantly male image-mongers of Western culture saturate the media with pictures of thin women contoured like perpetual adolescents, and ignore or degrade images of the traditionally, naturally plump female figure. If the male hatred of women has a tangible shape, it is that of the "perfect" woman with big breasts for feeding male fantasies and an otherwise anorexic shape that reflects a masculinized ideal. And while ours is a society that pays eager lip service to motherhood and pressures women to bear children, the consummate contempt for the "matronly" female shape so consistently associated with motherhood reveals volumes about the true American opinion of mothers. The message is loud, clear and insolent: women should assume the "mommy" role of taking care of everyone while putting their own needs last, but they should also look like slender, nubile child-women while they're doing it. Women ought to have babies or they're not "real" women, but they should also make damn sure they don't let it show on their bodies.

It has been said that beauty is the only type of power women have traditionally been able to exercise. But power that requires the imprimatur of others—and which is revoked by others when the beauty eventually fades—is second-hand power at best and a mere phantom compared to the status and respect that men typically command on the basis of what they accomplish, rather than what they look like. Male control of feminine imagery makes women malleable and docile by convincing them that they are never good enough as is, that they must always adhere to what they are taught is every man's desire, i.e., a slender body with large breasts, if they want sexual acknowledgement, approval and fulfillment.

Women, and especially fat women, are familiar with the unwavering and arrogant scorn with which men view women whose bodies fail to please the male eye. Male members of the Naval Academy, for example, reportedly have held contests for the ugliest date called "Pig Pushes," and keep what they call "Hog Logs" of the women (Burke, 1992). Understandably, the fear of ridicule intimidates many fat women into living lives of furtive appeasement. They may hide themselves from sight as much as possible, or obligingly wear clothes that carefully conceal their bodies; in short, apologizing for their failure to live up to the outrageous standards of sexiness which constitute such a large part of the feminine job description.

The Trickle-Down Effect: Weight Prejudice as Sexism Revisited

In a way, weight prejudice is the last bastion of sexism. It's been stated often enough that the burden of perpetual slenderness falls more heavily upon women's shoulders than men's, and that the penalties for "excess" weight are more severe for women than for men, a situation which, by itself, qualifies weight prejudice as inherently sexist. But there's more to it than that. Many of the most virulent stereotypes about women in general have not been discarded but merely transferred, so that negative qualities once attributed to all women are now considered the sole province of fat women.

For example, just as women entering the work force in the 1960's and 1970's had to confront scornful doubts about their abilities and dedication, just as they had to work twice as hard as men to get half the credit and recognition, now it is the heavy woman who often must fight battles simply to make it past an interviewer who assumes that fat women are uniformly slow, slovenly, and sick.

Just as all women were once faced with a culture that told them they were too emotionally unstable to be trusted with serious work, now it's fat women who are characterized as neurotic messes. And while society is no longer quite as quick to think of all women solely as mothers or mothers-to-be, it automatically assigns to the larger female shape the label of "motherly" or "matronly" while simultaneously desexualizing big women as sodden, passive lumps of flesh.

Whereas all women were once supposedly at the mercy of their hormones, now it is fat women who are seen as helpless pawns to their appetites for food. Whereas women as a group have had to struggle for the most basic respect and acknowledgement of their authenticity as individuals, now it is fat women who are faced with insistent stereotypes that label them as basically comical and/or pathetic, i.e., utterly unauthentic. And remember how unattractive, how unfeminine, a woman was considered to be when she was "aggressive"? Or, as Dr. Benjamin Spock wrote, "I believe women are designed in their deeper instincts to get more pleasure out of life...when they are not aggressive....when women are encouraged to be competitive too many of them become disagreeable." Compare Spock's opinion with this case history from *Doctor Schiff's Miracle Weight-Loss Guide*:

> *D.J. was a tall, "shocking" redhead. At 6'4" most of her excess pounds (she weighed 161) were on her legs and rear end. "She appeared to be a witch when she came in," recalls my nurse. "Too much black make-up on her eyes and a very loud voice." Two months later, D.J. had learned much about herself, thinking and writing. She had done*

some reprogramming. Now she was 17 pounds lighter, a more slender figure, wore less make-up and perfume, also her voice and manner were toned down and feminine (1974, p. 156).

In sum, at the same time that women were beginning to make progress against cultural assumptions of their inferiority, these same assumptions became part and parcel of the militantly negative popular image of fat women. It hardly seems a coincidence, then, that the definition of "fat" continues to become ever broader and encompass more women, while the most desirable body size continues to shrink; consequently, more women become convinced that they are fat and therefore inferior, and misogynists can conveniently disguise their politically incorrect disgust for women as a socially acceptable contempt for "unhealthy" fat.

A Woman's Dieting is Never Done

Feminists have frequently complained about the use of the words "man" and "mankind" to describe both men and women. It's still all too common to see the pronoun "he" employed even when it's clear that the persons referred to include females as well as males. Wouldn't it be nice if, just once, someone would use the female pronoun as a matter of course? Well, look no farther. A glance at the average diet-or weight-related newspaper or magazine article soon reveals that such articles almost always address women. There are no ambiguous collective pronouns in this arena.

Look at the ads for the different diet, exercise, and cosmetic surgery programs available. How many are aimed at women as opposed to men? One advertisement for plastic surgery, which asserts that "Beauty is more than skin deep," represents the results of the surgeon's handiwork as "perfection personified," and suggests that "[you] throw him a curve." In a book called *Beauty Surgery*, author William Canada, M.D. describes two different shapes of large women's hips as "riding breeches deformity" or "heavy buffalo type[s]" and a "violin deformity." In his section on abdominal surgery, he mostly discusses the operation as it pertains to women and the aftereffects of having children; no mention is made of the male tendency to develop beer bellies. Likewise, in the section entitled "Buttocks Reduction or Thigh Lift," all gender-specific references allude to women.

> *What's a surer giveaway of age than crow's feet? A flabby bottom....There is hardly a woman thirty-five or over who does not have flabby buttocks. As they pass you on the beach in a bikini or in the supermarket in slacks, the need for a buttocks lift is glaringly apparent....When changing fashion brings shorter skirts, the heavy buttocks are impossible to camouflage. Because of the inability to hide this problem, psychological problems related to poor body image may result. Look in any woman's magazine and the model is wearing close fitting clothes which reveal small, firm buttocks and thin thighs* (Canada, p. 118).

In another book on the subject, one set of before-and-after photos depict the work done on a "teenager who was self-conscious about the size of her hips and thighs" (Nemetz, 1988); the "before" picture displays an almost non-existent bulge on the girl's body. Clearly, even women with minuscule so-called flaws are all too willing to have their bodies slit open—generally by a man—so silicone "stuffing" can be inserted into some areas and fatty "stuffing" removed from others, as if they were dolls being reshaped. Where is the dignity in being a doll, in being coerced into not growing up or growing old? Beauty may lie in the eyes of the beholder, but it often seems as if fear and self-loathing lie in the eyes of the beheld.

One Weight Watchers' commercial not too long ago featured a woman saying she had tried "every diet known to *woman*." Once, when purchasing a box of diet shake powder, I noticed that all the pictures and advice on the back of the box referred exclusively to women. While we're at it, which gender of the human species comes complete with a natural extra layer of subcutaneous fat? Women. Which half of the human race, although until recently rarely the subjects of medical studies on heart disease and weight, is constantly being exhorted to dispose of all of its so-called extra fat? Women again. It's really very simple: dieting is women's work. Women, not men, are encouraged to define themselves as numbers: listen closely to women, even feminists, talk about their clothing sizes, and you will hear phrases like "I *am* a size 14," "I *was* a size 16," "I used to *be* a size 12," etc. A man takes, or needs, or wears a size; a woman *is* a size. Women, not men, constitute the majority of dieters. Women are more likely than men to think they have weight problems. Women are pressured to be perfect wives, perfect mothers, and perfect lovers with perfect bodies, in much the same way that men are pressured to be emotionally invulnerable moneymakers.

Fear and Loathing: Why Women Do It

Women have only recently begun to question society's latest demands on their bodies. It is my dear hope that future generations of women will look back on this era of frenzied dieting and cosmetic surgery with the same disgust and outrage with which enlightened women today view the old Chinese custom of footbinding, the African/Middle Eastern custom of genital mutilation, and the old American custom of steel corsets. But can we afford to wait for future generations? There's no doubt that some women are afraid of facing a vacuum of standards by which to judge themselves and each other if not by the weight scale and the tape measure.

Others, perhaps, are afraid to scratch the surface of their relationships, to scrutinize the motivations of family, friends and/or mates should they dare to break one of the most urgent social commandments of all to modern women: Thou shalt be thin. After all, since fat women are sometimes rejected as potential friends and mates, even used as scapegoats within their own families, purely because of their size, it is logical to assume the reverse is also true: that thin women are sometimes loved and accepted primarily or conditionally on the basis of their "good" looks, and it's hard to imagine many thin women wanting to confront this ugly human trait.

Weight can also serve as the focus of a power game between men and women, with husbands and lovers grumbling in a martyred manner about the "little woman" having "let herself go" and never letting her forget that she has not fulfilled her part of an unspoken bargain. It may be easier for her to play along with this nasty game than to risk defying other people's expectations, especially since this attitude is broadly reinforced by society. In a news article about divorced women, one woman related being dumped for gaining weight. Apparently, her ex-husband liked to taunt her by saying, "You could get diabetes and they'll cut your legs off right here." He would then pretend to saw off her legs (Hampson, 1992). A woman who steps beyond the boundaries of convention is quite likely to find herself an outsider, and we all know it.

Actually, it should come as no shock that women hesitate to challenge the dictatorial injunction to get and stay thin, nor should it surprise us that the women who oppose these dictates are treated as hypersensitive harpies and humorless shrews. Ridicule of social protest—and protesters—goes back a long way. The systemic harassment that comprises a large part of weight prejudice is similar to the sort of treatment inflicted upon the suffragettes of the 19th and early 20th centuries. Editorial cartoons often portrayed these extraordinary women as ugly, bitter, frustrated spinster types who were too unfeminine to have gotten a man and a family, like "real" women. Gladys and Marcella Thum, authors of *The Persuaders:*

Propaganda in War and Peace, comment upon the price the early suffragettes paid for their struggle to obtain the vote for women and the types of propaganda employed by their opponents:

> *The strongest device was the Appeal of Ridicule, the kind of humor that is used to cut an opponent "down to size" and make him—in this case, her—a figure of fun. The effectiveness of this propaganda can still be seen today. The women who fought for women's suffrage were some of the most respected and intelligent women of their day. So successful, however, was the prop-aganda of ridicule used against them, so widespread and merciless was it, that even to this day the picture of the "suffragette" and "feminist" is a caricature—an ugly, mannish figure, often in big bloomers and smoking a cigar—a figure of fun in the public mind.*
>
> *Out of this ridicule and its grotesque stereotype came fear. Any woman, and any man, too, fears being a figure of fun. Partly because of this fear, the suffragist movement progressed very slowly even after the vote was won* (Thum/Thum, 1972).

Plus ca change, plus c'est la meme chose. The more things change, the more they remain the same. The fact is that the deeply ingrained tyranny of weight prejudice is really just another way for a male-dominated culture to define women in terms expedient to the ruling class. This pernicious type of bullying crawls like a worm under a woman's skin and burrows its way to her heart, so that she must constantly struggle simply to be at peace with her own flesh, let alone enjoy its pleasures. But as long as women spend years of their lives and billions of dollars torturing themselves with diets, as long as they yearn wistfully for the promised magic of liposuction and the cosmetic surgeon's knife, or risk their health, even their lives with questionable diet pills and experimental weight-loss surgery, society raises no real objections. After all, this feminine *sturm und drang* reflects a strong urge to live up to traditional expectations and to please others. But let a woman relax, let her say to hell with diets, that she's fine just the way she is, and demand to be judged on her merits rather than on how close her measurements come to Barbie's, and instantly she becomes a slovenly rebel digging her grave with her fork.

> *Some fat people are even extolling the virtues, advantages, and benefits of being fat, claiming they are happier, more loved and loveable, sexually superior (with studies to prove it), of sweeter disposition, less moody, funnier, extroverted, et cetera, than those who carry fewer pounds. DON'T YOU BELIEVE IT! Those are fantasies, a* "fata morgana *(a mirage)."*
>
> Wiebe
> *3500 Calories=One Pound,* 1980

What more vulnerable spot to strike at in a woman than her physical self-image? What better way to make her and keep her insecure and desperate than to tell her she's ugly and undeserving of love, success, and happiness if her body weight exceeds a certain number of pounds? A TV actress unknowingly pointed out the problem when she said in an interview, "Oh, to be able to eat anything you want and still be loved" (Kitaen, 1992).

I remember reading a newspaper article about Naomi Wolf's powerful book, *The Beauty Myth*. The article described the basic precepts of the work, but also carefully pointed out from the start that Ms. Wolf is a beautiful woman (Kahn, 1991a). The tone implied that had Wolf been less than conventionally attractive, her credibility would have been open to question. In another instance, a local newspaper quoted rocker Courtney Love, "explaining her nose job, weight loss and dyed blond hair" as saying, "I want my anger to be valid, and the only way to do that is to be fairly attractive" (Love, 1995). In other words, a woman who actually suffers from the adverse effects of weight prejudice and who protests the attendant social injustice (which she is more than qualified to describe) cannot be taken seriously because she could only be a bitter, ugly loser who couldn't get herself a man—exactly like the ridiculed suffragettes described earlier.

With hindsight, of course, we realize that the early feminists were heroines, not bitter "losers," just as we know that the early African-American civil rights activists were not merely "jealous" because they couldn't sit at the front of the bus like whites or drink from the same water fountains. But the "sour grapes" line of reasoning is meant to keep victims of social injustice silent, ashamed, and invisible and, in the fat woman's case, to insinuate that any bias or harassment she experiences is either a normal response to her alleged inferiority or merely a by-product of her manifest jealousy and resentment.

Blindly obsessed with thinness, American society refuses to acknowledge that there is even a battle to be fought, let alone one in which a heavy woman is competent to engage. And instead of combating stereotypes, women often end up attacking themselves and each other, the "battle of the bulge" being a more acceptable preoccupation than uprooting comfortable assumptions.

> *But, one may ask, what if a man by his nature makes his life subservient to the images which he produces in others? Can he, in such a case, still become a man living from his being?... The widespread tendency to live from the recurrent impression one makes instead of from the steadiness of one's being is not a 'nature'....It is no light thing to be confirmed in one's being by others, and seeming deceptively offers itself as a help in this. To yield to seeming is man's essential cowardice, to resist it is his essential courage.*
>
> Martin Buber
> *The Knowledge of Man,* 1965

The Fat Woman as Anti-Status Symbol

Some big women do believe that their fat has one undisputable benefit: it protects them from sexual harassment and rape. This is true only to a certain extent. While a heavy female is unlikely to attract the attentions of immature, status-obsessed men who try to prove their masculinity by conquering thin beauties, and while a large percentage of men do treat big women as sexually invisible, weight prejudice nevertheless constitutes its own category of sexual harassment. Just because a woman does not conform to current standards of attractiveness does not mean that she is not considered a sexual object.

The only difference between a thin woman beheld as beautiful and one who is fat and thus perceived as ugly is that the first is considered a desirable commodity—i.e., someone who confers status on any lover with whom she is associated—while the other is treated like a *failed* sexual object, someone who stirs no envy or admiration in others. Just as the fat woman is consistently portrayed as an *anti*-role model for other women, she is also invariably represented as an *anti*-status/sex symbol for men.

In a 1972 comic strip drawn by *Mad Magazine*'s Dave Berg, a woman whose back is to the reader complains to a man about how men have dominated women and treated them as sex objects. In the last panel she turns around, angrily demanding that the man cease and desist this practice, but now the reader sees that she is a very heavy, coarse-featured older woman, and the man looks at her in utter astonishment. The offensive message here, which has not changed much in the last twenty years, is that this type of female is so unattractive that it is amusing that she could possibly consider herself the object of any form of male attention. In other words, female sexuality and a lack of "good" looks are mutually exclusive. This viewpoint defines a woman's sexual identity and value in terms of the adolescent, male perspective. By consistently drawing a sharp distinction between thin women and their heavier sisters, society reduces women to so many pieces of chocolate lined up in a candy box.

As for rape, unfortunately, no woman is exempt from the risk of this ultimate sexual violence. While the fat woman is probably not accused of "asking for it" by flaunting her supposedly non-existent charms, she may, incredibly, have to endure the world's wonderment at a rapist's selection of her as a victim. One heavy woman writing in to *Big Beautiful Woman* magazine recounted a hideous tale of being attacked by an intruder in her home one night and later calling the police, who didn't believe her story, only to overhear one officer ask the other, in apparent amazement, "Who would want to rape her?" (Anonymous, *BBW,* 1990) The idea that a fat woman is so repulsive that even a rapist demeans himself by touching one, is as sickening as sexist, and as hateful as weight prejudice can get.

Preference vs. Prejudice

In the Victorian marriage market, men judged and chose;
in the stakes of the beauty market, men judge and choose.
It is hard to love a jailer, women knew when they had no
legal rights. But it is not much easier to love a judge.
                    Naomi Wolf
                    The Beauty Myth

What does a fat woman see when she looks at men? Many undoubtedly see friends, lovers, and husbands. Others cannot. Some fat women, whose lives were or are filled with verbal abuse and sneering disregard, can only see judges and juries, tape measures with legs, merciless and unforgiving calculating machines. Some may see in men a consuming desire less for love, affection, and companionship than for the egotistical satisfaction that comes with possessing a "babe" with a great body.

In a newspaper article about the symbiotic relationships between male media stars and female fashion models, one rock star's manager simply admitted, "If you're free to go out with anybody, wouldn't your first choice be some gorgeous 21-year-old blonde, before it would be that sweet secretary down the hall with the thick behind?" (Warrick, 1992) Even the most sensitive man devoid of any overt machismo may unconsciously focus exclusively on thin women as potential romantic partners; they honestly think that their choices are purely coincidental, just an accident of circumstances, when in fact the cultural programming has gotten to them as well.

Men, of course, will reply that they simply have a preference for thin women, and who's to say they don't have that right? That's fine; but where weight and women are concerned, the line between preference and prejudice is razor-thin. The man who admits that he himself is not attracted to fat women, if he acknowledges that others may be, is expressing a subjective, if narrow-minded, opinion. But the man who, like the ones quoted below, suggests or states outright that *everyone* knows fat women are ugly and sloppy, and that no self-respecting man would touch one with a ten-foot pole, is striving to make of his subjective opinion an objective, undisputed fact. Strident inflexibility combined with contemptuous ridicule are dead giveaways of prejudice masquerading as a harmless partiality.

> *If you happen to be obese, resolve here and now that you're going to get rid of all those ugly pounds. With the proper diet and exercise, you can trim yourself down to where you won't be embarrassingly fat.*
>
> *It's a known fact that if you're a fat slob, your chances of meeting men are pretty slim. Obesity turns most men off. Unless you have a glandular disorder, this also indicates that you don't take much pride in your appearance.*
>
> Diebel
> *Finding Mr. Right: A Woman's Guide to Meeting Men,* 1990

In two separate newspaper articles about two different dating services, the owners and managers of these services all insisted that women don't really care about a man's height as much as the men do, or think the women do, but that men care deeply about a woman's weight—even if it is just a matter of ten pounds (Russo, 1991). Such men, one owner stated, would advise her after an arranged blind date that they had liked the woman but were nevertheless not interested in dating her again—solely because of her weight. The owner's attitude? "Women tend to underestimate the importance of overweight to their 'bondability....A woman will think 10 to 15 pounds isn't that much.'" (Kahn, 1992b) Naturally, neither article provided an opportunity for any of these "overweight" rejects to express *their* disappointment at being stuck with such fools. Where weight is involved, rejection is understood to be the thin person's sole prerogative, and a fat woman is considered a beggar, not a chooser.

Ironically, a third newspaper item about a matchmaking service between Russian women and American men included a remark from one man embittered by the women's preoccupation with his American citizenship and money rather than his personality, although the men in this service reportedly insist that the women be slender and conventionally attractive (Gransden, 1991). Clearly, men despise golddiggers who make their "love" conditional upon the size of a man's bank account; how odd, then, that men find it perfectly reasonable when a woman is accepted or rejected entirely on the basis of her face and figure, which are the feminine equivalent of "gold." American society must think it's acceptable as well, since we have no specific, established terms for this male version of gold-digging. Preference, then, is often just a euphemism for good old-fashioned sexist objectification of women.

A man raises status with other men by having a beautiful, wonderful woman on his arm....The worst thing a woman can do is the moment she's married, take the makeup off

and put the pounds on. It tells me she doesn't like herself
enough to take care of herself.
> From a news article about
> "single men today" and what
> they really want in a woman;
> Kato, 1991

Preferences, indeed. Notice how easily this man acknowledges that he admires women primarily not as individuals but rather for the status that their beauty confers upon him in the eyes of others; note, too, how casually he admits that a woman who ceases to serve this function (thus depriving him of his "top dog" status) lowers herself in his eyes. To him, it is the *woman's* disregard of her social obligations that constitutes the crux of the problem, the *woman's* transformation from a status symbol to a mere mortal that kills love and nullifies happiness. He accuses this hypothetical wife of not taking care of herself, but his real complaint is that she's not taking care of him and his macho, competitive needs.

Some people insist that women dress primarily to impress other women, but it is equally true that many men date and even marry to impress other men. When a man refuses to date any woman who is even 10 pounds "overweight," he is displaying not only a rigid bias but also a craven obedience to popular opinion. In fact, just as a great many gay people remain in the closet because they cannot endure the violent ridicule our culture imposes on them, it's quite likely that many men who privately admire the beauty of large women are hiding in their own closet because they have no wish to be mocked as freaks and failures by association.

Many FAs (Fat Admirers, or people who prefer partners
who are heavy) have a hard time accepting their
preference. Some of them live a life of denial where they
do not admit to themselves (or anyone else) that they
prefer a fat partner....One of the most frustrating things for
many FAs is the lack of acceptance among their peers.
Young FAs find it very hard to do "boys' talk" with their

friends for fear of being ridiculed. Many choose dates whom they do not find physically attractive (i.e., thin ones) just to please their buddies.

Blickenstorfer
"Survey of Male Fat Admirers"
NAAFA Workbook

Divide and Conquer: The Chick vs. The Pig

The contrast fostered between thin and heavy women reduces us all to the level of the barnyard and zoo. Chicks, hens, beavers, foxes, bitches—you name it, it has probably been used to describe a woman or her body. The fat woman is variously compared to a dog, a pig, a cow, a hippo or an elephant. She is not seen as human, and certainly not a bona fide female human. Weight prejudice, together with other aspects of appearance obsession, promotes competition between those women who can live up to the anorexic standards, whatever it takes, and those who cannot or will not. As a result, the fat woman has a two-pronged struggle on her hands: she must fight not only for equality with men but also for a level playing field with thin women. It's hard to say which is the more difficult endeavor.

But while this system is in place, the heavy woman not only must deal with the low social value assigned her, but also is forced to pay the price for the thin woman's superior status: she must suffer the indignities of invisibility so that the latter may stand out more distinctly as an object of admiration. A 1992 newspaper interview of comedian Richard Lewis included a recounting of his first meeting with a sexpot actress in an exercise spa. He began his story by describing two very heavy women who were working out, followed immediately by his impression of the thin actress when she walked in the door. At first glance, there seemed no reason for including the fat women in the story, but upon reflection it became obvious: the fat women served purely as a counterpoint to the tall, slender, blonde actress's stunning beauty. They were in the story *only* to provide contrast (Zehme, 1992). No wonder, then, that women contend so strenuously for attention and validation with their faces and figures. Just as men have traditionally established a pecking order on the basis of how many bucks and "babes" they can harvest, women similarly strive to attain the prizes that a "hot bod" can bring. Their physical measurements become a type of cultural currency that can open doors if the numbers are right, or slam them shut if they're wrong.

> *It is unthinkable that a woman bent on "having it all"*
> *would want to be fat, or even plump....*
> Helen Gurley Brown
> *Having It All,* 1982

What's worse, some women use these numbers not only to reap rewards from men but also to establish their dominance over other women. I can best illustrate this with a story a friend told me about a trip she made to a local chapter of a popular weight-loss program. As usual, she and the other women had lined up to be weighed one at a time by the counselor. One woman, who apparently had just recently achieved her "goal" weight, simply couldn't enjoy her triumph quietly. She came in wearing a swimsuit, and actually paraded back and forth before the other women standing in line, broadcasting her new-found superiority to the rest of them based on the numbers on the scale. The entire exchange was non-verbal and must have been about as subtle as an atomic bomb blast.

Of course, women, and especially "inferior" fat women, are never supposed to get angry at anyone but themselves. If others are cruel, they have only their own weakness to blame, so that the type of nasty power-tripping described above generally goes unchallenged. After all, if a so-called "plain" woman hates a gorgeous "babe," it couldn't be anything but jealousy, could it? Indeed, such jealousy is always presumed, even while the very real social injustice that fuels it is conveniently denied. In this way, the pecking order remains in place, unquestioned. It's funny how women think nothing of deriding men for trying to prove their masculinity with boorishly exaggerated, macho behavior. We forget that insecure thin women can also get caught up in the need to prove their femininity, often at the expense of those who are heavier. And what better way to do so than by flaunting a slender body?

> *I wanted people to look at me and see something special....From what I've seen, more people fail at losing weight than at any other single goal. I found out how to do what everyone else couldn't: I could lose as much or as little weight as I wanted. And that meant I was better than everyone else* (Sacker and Zimmer, 1987).

> *'It was about power,' says Kim Morgan, speaking of her obsession with slenderness, 'that was the big thing...something I could throw in people's faces, and they would look at me and I'd only weigh this much, but I was strong and in control, and hey **you're** sloppy...'* (Bordo, 1985)

I recall watching a talk show featuring very heavy men and women as the guests. A thin woman in the audience who was clearly upset and close to tears announced that she had recently lost a considerable amount of weight. Why, she wondered, should she have gone to so much trouble if fat people succeeded in attaining equal social status? She seemed to feel that her accomplishment would in some way be diminished if that were to happen. In effect, what she was saying was that her entry into acceptable society was not meaningful unless she could continue to compare herself favorably to, and at the expense of, bigger women. *Her self-esteem relied in significant part upon the self-hatred and inferior status of fat women.* It reminded me of an old *Peanuts* comic strip in which one character, a little girl, asks other little girls if they're jealous of her because she has naturally curly hair. When they reply no, they're not jealous, that they're satisfied with themselves just as they are, she is disappointed, and walks away saying, "What's the good of having naturally curly hair if nobody's jealous?" (Schulz, 1969) What, indeed? Would women still pursue thinness with the same sense of urgency if they could not derive an artificial, illusory sense of superiority from the distinction?

Weight prejudice divides women between the so-called "winners" and "losers" and sets us at each other's throats. How many times have we heard, or said ourselves, "She's so thin. Don't you just hate her?" or "Couldn't you just kill her?" How often have we heard the words "anorexic" or "bulimic" used as an insult to describe very skinny women, even though true anorexia or bulimia reflects terrible suffering, even a rejection of life? Nevertheless, whatever her true physical and emotional state may be, the thin woman is automatically commended for her willpower, her sexiness, her vibrant health, and her overall superior value in American society. The slender figure is hysterically celebrated and coveted.

And the rest of us? We are persuaded that women only come in two sizes: very thin or too big, and we're probably the latter. Whoever turns her back on this relentless beauty contest is seen as a slob who doesn't "like herself enough to take care of herself" or a bitter man-hater who will never be a "real" woman. Shulamith Firestone says it well in *The Dialectic of Sex: The Case for Feminist Revolution*:

> *Every society has promoted a certain ideal of beauty over all others. What that ideal is is unimportant, for any ideal leaves the majority out; ideals, by definition, are modeled on rare qualities....If and when, by artificial methods, the majority can squeeze into the ideal, the ideal changes. If it were attainable, what good would it be?*
>
> *For the exclusivity of the beauty ideal serves a clear political function. Someone—most women—will be left out. And left scrambling, because as we have seen, women have been allowed to achieve individuality only through*

*their appearance—looks being defined as "good" not out of
love for the bearer, but because of her more or less
successful approximation to an external standard....If they
don't, the penalties are enormous: their social legitimacy is
at stake* (1970, p. 152).

Unfortunately, even though American society is finally tuning in
to the damage caused by weight/body obsession, the discussion
usually focuses on the pain suffered by thin and medium-sized
women in the forms of anorexia and bulimia. Women in these size
groups are discouraged from thinking of themselves as fat when they
are not, yet the underlying message remains the same—that fat is
bad and ugly. Thus, "normal" sized women are gathered back into
the social fold, while big women remain out in the cold, and society
can conveniently continue to ignore the latter, who are *still*
invisible—even when the subject is weight obsession.

If women are to break through this artificial wall which so often
results in bitter rivalry and animosity, we must divest ourselves of
two popular and deeply entrenched fantasies: first, that fat women
are invariably ugly, loveless losers, and second, that all thin women
are by comparison paragons of perfection who lead, or at least
deserve to lead, successful lives free of trouble or strife. Female
weight bigots need to examine with a critical eye their narrow
definition of beauty and accept the plump figure as just one variation
on a theme rather than a fate worse than death or a negation of
femininity. At the same time, big women who have bought the
overwrought lies of the mainstream culture need to disengage
themselves from the psychological tricks and traps designed to keep
them invisible.

Thinness = Happiness: Fantasy vs. Fact

ITEM: California. July 2, 1995. Would-be supermodel Krissy Taylor dies at the age of 17 of respiratory problems. Heart failure brought on by use of a bronchial spray is suspected.

ITEM: California. April 14, 1989. Ramon Salcido murders his wife (a beautiful, thin model), his mother-in-law, his sister-in-law, and two of his three young daughters, in a bloody rampage.

ITEM: 1992. *TV Guide* "Grapevine" advertises a TV-movie about a former Miss America who was abused by her ex-fiance.

ITEM: 1991. Former beauty queen Miss Georgia, Frances Frazier, dies at the age of 28 from a heart condition which included a partially clogged coronary artery.

ITEM: California. April, 1991. Twenty-three-year-old Jennifer Lilly—tall, thin, blonde, and beautiful—is brutally murdered by her estranged ex-boyfriend.

ITEM: California. 1986. Slender, attractive Renee June is missing together with her baby daughter and presumed dead. Her ex-husband, the prime suspect, later commits suicide.

ITEM: San Diego, California. 1989. Formerly "blond and sleek" Elisabeth Anne Broderick murders her ex-husband and his new wife, another slender blonde. Broderick recounts a tale of a miserable marriage.

These items illustrate, in a manner that mere opinion cannot, that the thin woman does not always live happily ever after. While a slender body often assures a woman of more and better economic and/or social opportunities than a full figure, it is not a guarantee of happiness, love, self-esteem, good health, long life, or success, no matter how desperately society promotes that fantasy.

Unfortunately, there are fat women, many of them veteran yo-yo dieters, who are so mesmerized by the alluring promises made by the diet industry and so convinced that a thin body is the path to an earthly Paradise, that they would be at a loss to understand that a thin woman might have problems. But if we set aside for a moment all the deceitful mass media images we see, we will realize that few, if any, of the thin women we know are rich and famous, nor are they covered with adoring men, perfectly healthy, permanently young, or endowed with infinite talent, humor, self-esteem, ambition and charm. Thin females are no more immune to violence, child abuse, sexual harassment, loneliness, disease, neurosis, psychosis, and untimely death than anyone else.

Certainly, the advice columns in the newspapers are never at a loss for letters from distraught women in a variety of unhappy situations, and it hardly seems likely that they are all heavy women. Nor is it remotely possible that every woman who has ever been abused, rejected, deceived, betrayed, or abandoned by a man is a large woman. If this seems overly harsh, let us keep in mind the relentlessly hostile and negative picture that society typically paints of the large woman, her character, and her destiny. Let us remember, too, that people often question the credibility of a man enamored of a fat woman, and his motivations are brought under a suspicious, puzzled scrutiny. Moreover, a big woman is generally expected to assume that any man who would find her attractive must have something wrong with him.

> ...you ought to be suspicious of men who say they like fat **women**. Those men want **mothers**, or at least a comfy, cushiony, sofa-pillow girl to sink into and hide out in.
> Helen Gurley Brown
> *Having It All,* 1982

The fate of most bone-thin actresses and models should be a lesson to all females on the disposability of the pretty woman: one year they are held up before us as mortal goddesses and the next they are treated as parched, passé has-beens. It's hard to say which is worse, a cultural order that views women as toys to be played with and discarded when they're worn out, or a woman who means to gain something from this system and knowingly collaborates, regardless of the price she and other women will pay for her accidental (or surgically acquired) good looks. But if conventional beauty really is the most valuable asset a woman can possess, and if individual qualities like intelligence, personality, compassion, etc., are truly of no consequence, then the slender, pretty woman is little more than an interchangeable cog in the wheel of male desires and social expectations.

Certainly, if the lives of women like Elizabeth Taylor and Marilyn Monroe or, more recently, the English Princess Diana teach the rest of us anything, it is that being a sex goddess or a world-renowned regal beauty is no guarantee of emotional security, fulfillment, good health, fairy-tale love, or even simple contentment. Unfortunately, millions of women in America continue their wild-goose chase of anorexic chic, foolishly thinking that it will unlock the secrets of happiness and unconditional approval. Meanwhile, Hollywood and the mass media continue to feed people this fantasy as fast as they can swallow it.

Breaches of Privacy

Another component of the negative visibility that plagues almost every fat woman, and which reflects society's image of women as public property, is lack of privacy. When a person, whether stranger or intimate, comments on what a heavy woman is eating or on her appetite, that is a breach of privacy. When someone pokes a heavy woman's body or pinches her fat, that is a breach of privacy. When unsolicited diet and exercise advice is thrust upon a fat woman under the assumption that she could not possibly like herself as she is, that is a gross invasion of privacy. The size of a woman's body is no more anyone else's business than the size of her bank account, the contents of her dreams, or any other personal aspect of her life.

The irony in this situation is that, as we've already seen, heavy women are often considered by the so-called experts to be suffering from "boundary" problems; that is, they supposedly bury themselves in fat both to avoid the anxiety of competing with other women as well as to keep people at a distance (Zerbe, 1995). Let us assume, for the sake of argument, that this is true for *some* large women. In the first place, without the framework of weight prejudice, in a society that unreservedly accepted big women, this strategy would fail utterly. It is not possible, after all, to hide from the whole world unless the world cooperates by expecting you to get out of sight and doing its best to see that you stay there. In *The Body Betrayed,* Kathryn Zerbe, M.D., naively suggests that "Their ("obese" individuals) tendency to view thin as good and fat as bad must give way to a more integrated and less rigid view of self and others" (1995, p. 305). It hardly requires an M.D. to realize that this is a perfect description not of "obese individuals" but rather of weight bigots in particular and American society in general; when fat people hold such views, it is primarily because the principles of thin-is-good-and-fat-is-bad have been hammered mercilessly into their skulls since childhood. Zerbe's assertion only serves to support the cultural delusion that fat people exist in a social vacuum where they perpetuate their own problems.

In the second place, the invisible woman cannot truly hide as long as she is expected to reappear at society's whim to serve in her function as scapegoat. As a result, she must often endure assaults upon her "personal space" by family members, friends, and even total strangers who have very firm ideas about how she should eat and drink, look and feel, and why she is unwilling or unable to conform to popular standards. Although these meddlers will sweetly proclaim that the fat woman "owes it to herself" to become thin, what they really mean is that she owes it to them and their intrusive need to control her. It is they who lack an understanding of or respect for boundaries, they who insinuate themselves and their own prejudices and anxieties into the minds, hearts, and bodies of big people in order to fulfill their own personal or commercial agendas.

An integral part of 20th-century feminism has focused on the exclusive right of women to control their own bodies. But too often, even feminists have failed to understand that weight-related prejudice and obsession, like anti-abortion laws, hijack a woman's sense of physical privacy while appropriating her body and soul. How many pro-choice women who would never allow themselves to be coerced into an inappropriate reproductive choice, will permit cultural pressures to shape their eating patterns and body image? If the highest court in the land will uphold a woman's right to privacy as it relates to the issue of abortion, what gives bigots the right to demand that a woman constantly answer for her body size?

The subject of weight as it relates to beauty and personal worth is such a touchy matter for most women that few are willing to challenge the status quo on their own, and this is exactly why weight prejudice must be dragged out into the light of day and examined. The fine feminist fury that struggles to bring down patriarchal prejudices often seems to skid to a sheepish stop when brought face to face with the topics of body size and physical attractiveness. Even Gloria Steinem has written, in an article about women and self-image, "How many of us, for example, see ourselves as fat or otherwise unappealing, regardless of what our scales and mirrors tell us?" (1992) The fight for the right to control one's body in a reproductive context seems painfully contradictory when women continue to abdicate their right to physical self-determination every day at the dinner table.

Also, the disgusting number of crimes against women—sexual harassment, incest, molestation, and rape—proves irrefutably that a large number of men on some level perceive women's bodies as public display items presented for their pleasure, entertainment, criticism and casual use. What's worse, the fat woman must carry her so-called deviation out in the open, because, unlike some gay people, she has no closet in which to hide; she cannot try to "pass" for a "normal" person.

Americans have a bizarre, almost voyeuristic, fascination with other people's weight, and especially the weight gains and losses of public figures. Elizabeth Taylor, Roseanne, and Oprah Winfrey, to name just a few, have consistently been subjected to an intense and invasive scrutiny of their measurements. Many large women who are not famous can also speak with authority of encounters with people they have never seen before—and presumably will never want to see again—who think nothing of staring, pointing, or making snide remarks in passing, even asking a large woman who happens to be eating, "Do you really think you should be eating that?" or "You don't really need that, you know."

I once dined at a natural foods restaurant in Berkeley where two extremely thin and pinched-looking women in a nearby booth scrutinized my plate of vegetarian nachos with unmistakeable health-conscious horror mixed, I thought, with more than a touch of envy. I heard shocked, whispered murmurs of "cheese" and "so much fat" while my friend and I ate our meals. Imagine their consternation when I ordered a piece of carrot cake for dessert! Again, in such situations large women are visible only to be criticized and condemned. They are seen not as real people living real lives—and entitled to eat real food—but rather as undisciplined slobs who are not "PC" (physically correct). If such an outrageous disregard for her personal boundaries contributes to a feeling of paranoia in a heavy woman, it is no wonder.

Feeding issues are often a mask for power struggles between parent and child. When an adult examines and criticizes a daughter's every bite (What have you got there? What are you eating? How much did you take? You can't have a second helping!), the adult communicates a coarse disrespect for the child's privacy, in effect telling her that she cannot be trusted with her own body. This same dynamic can also be found in many adult relationships. One woman writing to Ann Landers' advice column asked for help concerning her son-in-law, who brought a weight scale on a family trip and threatened his wife with divorce if she ate a baked potato (Landers, 1992a).

Clearly, men and women still have a long way to go in learning how to perceive one another as individuals rather than types and objects, and we've seen how easily people slip into the lazy, sloppy habit of measuring women according to their shape and size. It's true, of course, that women are not morally pure, either. We often judge one another by the degree to which we have conformed to cultural expectations, and we are not exempt from appraising men on the basis of their height, weight, hairline or financial success; men, meanwhile, are still actively encouraged to value women for the high status accorded a slender body—a modern dowry, as it were. Bodies, money, beauty, success...the only difference is the terms on which the game is played. We all hope and wish to be valued and loved for ourselves, but our panicked, conformist behavior reflects the bitter fear that such acceptance is an impossible dream. And as long as these fears of rejection consume us, as long as people will believe anything, do anything, buy anything to win the game, the game will go on unchanged, with very few real winners, and with the fat woman pushed off to the sidelines, unwelcome and unseen.

CHAPTER FIVE

Food, Sex, and Power

The Invisible Woman
and the New Puritanism

Not to enjoy food is to reject life itself.
                    Ann Lee Harris
                    San Francisco restaurateur

"*E*verything enjoyable is either illegal, immoral, or fattening," the saying goes. What does it reveal about the American attitude toward food that "fattening" would end up alongside "illegal" and "immoral?" For one thing, it demonstrates that eating certain kinds of foods, like hot-fudge sundaes or deep-dish pizzas, has been accorded the status of a guilty pleasure somewhere on the darker side of human desires. Also, since the concepts of "illegal" and "immoral" have always embraced certain socially unacceptable sexual practices, we can see that Americans relate to "pleasure" foods with the same deep-seated conflicts generally associated with sex, such as craving versus control and individual desires versus social proscriptions. When a dieter eats "forbidden" food, she's said to be "cheating," a word with clear moral implications.

Glance through a newspaper and you'll probably encounter ads like the one for a fat-free cake mix that says, "No Fat. No Cholesterol. No Guilt." Guilt for what? Is it a crime to eat a piece of cake? Has a mortal sin been committed? Of course not, but women have been taught that any eating for pleasure is shameful, even a potential threat to their sexual viability. They are trained from a young age to feel contrite for consuming delicious food, ineffectual for eating three full meals a day, guilty for not exercising until they are perfectly toned. And when women break the rules, when their bodies—for whatever reason—exceed the narrow boundaries permitted by society, they run head-on into America's new puritanism.

> *Tolerance is not really being enlarged: it is moving its targets....Anyone who succumbs to alcoholism meets with less censure and more compassion than formerly ("it's an illness, really...perfectly understandable, the pressures are too great...."), but anyone who succumbs to obesity gets short shrift ("no excuse for it these days....only needs a bit of will power....**other** people manage not to let themselves go...."). The total number of moral attitudes struck, the difficulty of trying to conform to them, and the weight of social disapproval visited on those who fail vary hardly at all.*
>
> Elaine Morgan
> *The Descent of Woman,* 1972

The Eleventh Commandment: Thou Shalt Not Eat

The big woman especially finds herself caught in the cross-fire between America's cultural conflicts about food and sex. Instead of the intact hymen, society now uses numbers on the tape measure and weight scale as symbols of virtue or sin by which to measure femininity, respectability, and status, and to keep unruly feminine appetites in line. While "sexy" sin is in, it's now considered acceptable to look down upon a woman's appetite for food as a neurotic, even infantile, compulsion.

> *A 35-year-old woman who confesses to having an extramarital affair with a younger man says, "Exercise makes me a better wife, mother and lover, plus occasionally I get to eat something sinful," she said. She says she doesn't feel guilty about the affair; it's indulgence in food that troubles her* (Rubenstein, 1992).

> *Taking your body from lumpy to lithe can be daunting, especially when your efforts are played out on the public stage of the local gym....fitness fashion can cover up a multitude of sins—or expose a bod that's simply sinful* ("No-Sweat Style," Ragel, *TV Guide* 1994).

As a result, it is the fat woman who bears the brunt of this latest cultural taboo. Since sex is glorified and eating disparaged, the equivalent attitudes extend to the people whom society decides are engaging in these respective activities. A popular picture thus emerges that paints thin women as self-disciplined, fully sexual beings who either struggle nobly with their ignominious food-related appetites or who have little or no interest in the subject, while big women are characterized as preoccupied gluttons constantly eating and overeating at the expense of their sexual lives:

> *I wish more overweight women would be motivated to lose weight for (sexual affairs), but very few men want to start one with a fat woman. There will always be the occasional furtive one-night stands, as long as he doesn't have to exhibit her in public. But no flowers, diamonds, mink, and Caribbean vacations—they go to the thin girls. The overweight girls themselves are partly to blame; they do not send out sexual messages....The majority of single overweight women, I'm afraid, have settled for oral*

gratification, and sacrificed their sex lives to the pleasures of eating.

Edelstein
*The Woman Doctor's Diet
for Women,* 1977

Once again, the slender figure is put on a pedestal, while the big woman is seen not as an authentic woman on an equal sexual footing with other women, but rather as the collective, visible personification of excess.

Sex is commercially geared to the thin of thigh and the lean of heart.

Richard Simmons
Never-Say-Diet, 1980

The Food-Sex Double Standard

One of the accusations most frequently leveled at heavy people is that they become fat as a result of eating for all the wrong reasons; e.g., from boredom, from habit, or to soothe themselves in stressful situations. This argument is consistently used to distinguish the fat from the thin:

Instead of eating when your body tells you to—as animals do—you eat by the clock, or on command of others (parents, spouse, dinner companion, TV commercial) or when you emotionally feel you need balm and solace (when lonely, bored, frustrated, angry, depressed).

In other words, you eat on signal from external sources in your environment rather than from internal signals in your body.

Berland
The Dieter's Almanac, 1984

Let us assume, for the moment and purely for the sake of argument, that weight bigots are correct: that thin people are the primary participants in sexual activity while big people are mostly celibate hermits who sit on life's sidelines and eat. Since thin people are presumed to be such paragons of virtuous self-discipline, it would logically follow that this genius for rational control would be reflected in our society's patterns of sexual behavior. This is a supposition so absurd it's laughable. The truth is that human beings engage in sex for the same "wrong" reasons that they eat.

Indeed, in Desmond Morris' book *The Human Zoo* (1971), he devotes a chapter to what he terms "Sex and Super-Sex," in which he identifies no fewer than ten categories of human sexual motivation: Procreation Sex, Pair-formation Sex, Pair-maintenance Sex, Physiological Sex, Exploratory Sex, Self-rewarding Sex ("sex for sex's sake"), Occupational Sex, Tranquillizing Sex, Commercial Sex, and Status Sex. His explanations of "Occupational Sex" and "Tranquillizing Sex" are especially illuminating. He refers to the former as "an anti-boredom device" which "functions as a therapeutic remedy for the negative condition produced by a sterile and monotonous environment" (p. 85), and the latter as "anti-turmoil", something "similar to the animal activity known as 'displacement activity'" engaged in to "provide a momentary respite from the stressed condition" (pp. 87, 88).

In other words, people—and remember, we're only talking about thin people now—are prone to have sex because they're bored or for temporary comfort in response to stress. So much, then, for the emotional "flaws" peculiar to the so-called overeater. Apparently, vulnerability to displacement activity is unrelated to one's physical measurements.

Morris postulates further, "It is, after all, possible to indulge oneself gastronomically without growing either fat or sick. With sex the trick is more difficult to accomplish, and society is littered with the bitter jealousies, forlorn heartbreaks, miserable, shattered families and unwanted offspring to prove it" (p. 108). Morris also discusses the long-term, global consequences of sex without effective contraception, and his warning that unchecked population growth could lead to "the total collapse of the whole of human society" (p. 75) puts the potential repercussions of eating for reasons other than sheer survival into their proper perspective when compared to worldwide catastrophe.

As for "commercial sex," which Morris describes as "a milder form of sex-for-material-gain...executed by strip-teasers, dance hostesses, beauty queens, club girls, dancers, models and many actresses," a quick glance around us will confirm that American society is inundated with this particular expression of sexuality. Finally, "status sex" is not only cynical but has a tremendous potential for exploitation by either men or women:

> *Status Sex is concerned with dominance, not with reproduction....A male can copulate with a female primarily to boost his masculine ego, rather than to achieve any of the other nine sexual goals....The male who uses females for Status Sex purposes is more concerned, in fact, with showing them off than with anything else....* (pp. 90, 101, 102).

Of course, in our relentlessly sex-obsessed culture, the mere suggestion that (thin) people can and do become sloppy slaves to their hormones invites accusations of sexual repression. However, statistics show that approximately half of the 25.4 million pregnancies in the U.S. between 1984 and 1988 were unplanned (Bouvier/Grant, 1994), while other data reflect a rate of infection for sexually transmitted diseases standing at 12 million cases each year (Cowley/Hager, 1991). Taken together, these figures reflect an abundant overindulgence in sex for its own sake, sex for comfort or pleasure only, pure ego-satisfaction, out of habit or a sense of obligation, even as an expression of neurotic need, and without due consideration for the potential consequences. Nor need one be an expert to know that people often stay in otherwise bad relationships, sabotage good relationships, and take foolish risks merely to satisfy sexual desires.

> *In explaining why women sometimes fail to protect themselves and others after getting their (AIDS) test results, sociologists Jane Zones and Diane Beeson say that some women they studied interpreted their reassuring test results to mean that since they weren't already infected, they weren't going to be infected later. Others, they say, "had a mystical thing: They believed if they thought positively, they wouldn't get infected." For the majority, the researchers say, "it was just passion. People were so overcome with sexual feelings that they couldn't think."*
>
> Krajick
> "Private Passions & Public Health," *Psychology Today,* 1988

Where, then, are the derisive media images of these slender sexual hedonists and opportunists as lazy, weak, unattractive, demoralized slobs? Where is the daily, institutionalized ridicule of and discrimination against men and women—all of them thin, of course—who engage in irresponsible, unsafe, and/or meaningless sex purely to assuage personal insecurities, console themselves, stave off boredom or boost their egos and validate their sexual identities? Where are the bookshelves groaning under the weight of self-help volumes written to persuade the slender that they are physically and/or emotionally disturbed? That they must not live to have sex but instead have sex only to give life? Surely it's just a matter of willpower to avoid the risks incurred by "compulsive" sex. Surely these thin people realize that they're digging their graves with their sexual organs! Obviously, even the true overeater is hardly alone in her ability to stretch physical appetites to cope with all sorts of social and emotional needs and circumstances. And before American society points its self-righteous finger at the full-figured, it should first take a long look in the nearest mirror.

The Male-Female Double Standard

Then there's the other great American double standard about male and female appetites which has yet to go out of fashion. Just as sexual impulses have typically been something a man enjoyed but a woman controlled, today a big man with an unapologetic taste for food is perceived as hearty, robust, and somehow larger than life, while any big woman who possesses an uninhibited fondness for good food is disparaged as a compulsive slob.

> *Gerard Depardieu (a heavyset French actor) was famished....Instantly, three sous-chefs were busy cutting French bread into elegant slices, toasting them, and then...garnished them with a rich and thoroughly decadent layer of* foie gras. *Soon (Depardieu) was standing in the middle of the kitchen, drinking his wine, wolfing down foie gras, and making jokes with the sous-chefs and busboys. The scene was typical Depardieu....By nature, he is a gregarious peasant, with a peasant's appetites....He brings this same unbridled gusto and lack of pretense to the craft of acting....What Depardieu embodies...is raw animal magnetism—call it sex appeal, if you prefer....*
>
> Chutkow
> "The Peasant King," 1994

Women, of course, are not popularly admired for their physical appetites, only their denial of them. A woman is rewarded for self-deprivation—witness the praise and emotional support a dieting woman typically elicits merely by announcing her intentions—but a man is envied and admired for his lusts and cravings. Women simply aren't supposed to get hungry; it's not feminine, and certainly not attractive. In fact, one psychological study investigating the connection between a woman's social appeal and her eating habits found that women are rated as most feminine when they eat small salads, and least feminine when they eat heartier meals like meatball subs with fries and milkshakes (McAllister Smart, 1995). Not only are women supposed to be magically satisfied with child-sized portions of food, but they are also asked to choose between love or food, and not to be so greedy as to feel they deserve both.

Sadly, just as the male establishment has created and exploited this double standard as a means of keeping women anxious and dissatisfied with themselves, the slender woman often plays her own version of this game, only with herself as the one entitled to physical appetites while despising those of the fat woman as unnatural. Weight prejudice is partly a result of the "normal" woman's frustration and anxiety, as Charles Roy Schroeder eloquently explains in *Fat Is Not A Four-Letter Word,*

> *Losing an unnatural amount of body fat is an agonizing experience; keeping it off is a chronically agonizing experience....these miserable feelings may explain why thin women often have such hostile emotions toward fat women—particularly when the latter are happy with themselves and their lives....A woman who elects to chronically suffer from food deprivation and who regularly exercises to exhaustion to conform to public standards of thinness is understandably not eager to hear that fat women are in reality just as beautiful...it must be a bitter pill for the thin woman whose suffering has not made her happier at all* (1992, pp. 101-102).

It is therefore not surprising that the thin woman who clings to the idea that measurements are destiny would play along with the current system, since it both validates her own femininity and seeks to eliminate the big woman as a competitor in all walks of life. Indeed, even the thin woman who finds weight prejudice offensive and does not participate in it nevertheless stands to benefit from its continued practice. Certainly, the slender conformist who tortures herself in order to catch and keep a man's attentions doesn't want any more rivals than she has already. Also, since she has been taught, and is pleased to believe, that sexuality and a full figure are entirely incompatible, she is just as reluctant as her sexist male counterpart to let big women get away with enjoying either food or sex, let alone both, since she herself feels so caged-up and restricted.

> *I'm having dinner at a see-and-be-seen kind of place in the city with my costumer, Richard....The two thirtysomething women next to me can barely contain their horror as I clumsily try to pass through the space between our tables to slide onto the banquette seat....(They) are glaring at me. I order a goat-cheese salad and pasta with cream sauce. They giggle. The rest of the meal proceeds in much the same manner....I excuse myself to go to the ladies' room....Richard...tells me that as soon as I left, one of them asked him, "What are you doing with that fat pig?" He replied, "She's my girlfriend." "That's not possible," said one woman. "You must be a hustler."*
>
> Leslie Lampert
> "Fat Like Me," 1993

Sex, Food, and Love:
Short-Circuiting Primal Instincts

Although the weight-loss establishment promotes the fantasy that thin Americans are "above" any messy emotional ties to food, in fact we are all surrounded every day by associations between food, love, and sexuality, perhaps the most constant of which is our society's never-ending obsession with the female breast. Men and women alike still often equate a woman's bust size with the degree of her femininity, even though there is no objective connection. As a result, what is biologically a method for feeding infants becomes an overemphasized item of attraction for many men and a source of endless anxiety for many women.

It is not surprising, then, that breasts are the *only* female body parts which are popularly considered more attractive with increasing size. It's also hard to escape the fact that the physical feature most consistently celebrated in woman is that which feeds others. This attitude, combined with the more recent emphasis on a female physique that's tiny except in the chest, illuminates the cultural expectation that women provide others with boundless physical and psychological nurturing and pleasure while keeping their own needs and desires on a short, tight leash.

Most of us are aware, if only unconsciously, of the intimate relationship between the language of sex and the language of food. An attractive woman has been called a "dish," a "peach," or a "hot tomato." She may be referred to as "luscious" or "delicious," or, in some old movies, as a "cookie." Her complexion may be described as "peaches and cream." Her breasts may be compared to two scoops of ice cream or melons; her hymen is sometimes called her "cherry" and her lips often compared to the same fruit. She may look good enough to eat; and when a person says, "I could just eat you up," that is a signal of desire or affection. Oral sex is often referred to as "eating." A slang term for penetration is "hide the salami" and, for the penis, "pork sword;" thus, a man having sex is "porking" his partner or "feeding [a woman's] box." A man masturbating is "slapping the salami" or "beating the meat," and a man ejaculating is "creaming." When I was a child, we often referred to a boy's penis as a wiener or a hot dog.

Every respectable sex novelty shop carries a variety of flavored oils that can be licked off one's partner, as well as that all-time crowd-pleaser, edible underwear. And how many nights of romance are preceded by a delicious dinner? Licking and sucking are actions employed in both eating and lovemaking, although where food is concerned it is usually sweets, like candy or ice cream—"naughty" foods—that are consumed in such a fashion. One may be "starved" for love just as easily as for food. A person may refer to a loved one as "sweetheart," "sweetie pie," "sugar," "honey," "cupcake," etc.

Feminine beauty is sometimes referred to as "cheesecake" and the male equivalent, "beefcake." Sex is cutely termed "dessert."

The commercial world takes full advantage of the food-sex/love connection. Certain foods, like chocolate, have long been associated with romance and sexuality. We have Hershey's Kisses and Hugs. We have Almond Joy. Of course, although larger sizes in food products are often marketed as "King Size," have you ever seen a "Queen Size" candy bar or bag of sweets? Only in mattresses or pantyhose—*not* in foods. One ad for York Mint Patties displays a wrapper with the words, "Get the sensation!", while a pitch for margarine suggests that we "spread a little love" by spreading around the product. A layout for New Cool Whip Chocolate trumpets that it's "The *NEW* way to love chocolate," while Hershey puddings are touted as "Two Great Ways to Love Your Chocolate." A TV spot for Dove Silk features a thin woman dressed in silk emerging with a come-hither look from silken draperies. Yet another ad, for Pet-Ritz Pie Crusts, exhorts women to "Show your love," presumably by baking a pie. We see one advertisement after another before Valentine's Day urging people to express their affection with confections; "Don't Let Love Pass You By," says one such ad for Godiva chocolates; "Better Than Sex?!" chocolate cake, trumpets another for a sweet shop. Häagen Dazs Frozen Yogurt ads once featured a tall, thin blonde woman in a white bathing suit eating the product in a very sensual way. The slogan at the end of the commercial: Taste the Passion.

What, then, does the food-sex relationship mean for the fat woman? Just this: although she is surrounded by cues that reflect a healthy and normal association between two natural sources of pleasure, she is expected to short-circuit this primal connection. It's not so much that large women are supposed to forego food altogether—God knows, they can eat as much cottage cheese, small green salads and other diet foods as they like—but rather that they are expected to deprive themselves of the designated "pleasure" foods, such as chocolate, other sweets and any foods associated with love, sex, sin, and guilt. I remember seeing a couple walking ahead of me in a department store approach the candy counter on their left. When the woman started to veer toward it, her male companion firmly pulled her away, telling her, "*You* don't want that."

Nevertheless, a thin woman can be smothered in sweets from her sweetie and expect no repercussions as long as she keeps her figure. Naturally, every ad for sweets using romance as the hook depicts a thin woman as the recipient. The slender woman who responds to stress with a pint of ice cream is not perceived as neurotic unless she gains weight, but a fat woman who behaves similarly—even if such behavior occurs no more frequently than in her thin counterpart—is diagnosed as a compulsive overeater. In fact, many of the weight-loss preachers like to pretend that big people are the exclusive consumers of "naughty" foods.

> *Ever notice how fat people still eat the food little children are attracted to? Twinkies, cupcakes, ice cream, pizza, soda pop, macaroni and cheese, hot dogs, fudge, candy, mashed potatoes, french fries, hamburgers—ugh! If you are an adult person, your tastes should have changed somewhat by now.*
> Chapian and Coyle
> *Free To Be Thin,* 1979

Fat women are instructed to approach "pleasure" foods as they would a dark alley in the worst part of town, as the weight-loss hucksters self-righteously intone the motto, "Eat to live, don't live to eat." In our weight-prejudiced culture, partaking of "sexual" foods—like sex itself—is viewed as the exclusive privilege of thin people, even though society also pretends that thin people are either not eating these foods at all or at most indulge rarely.

At the same time, the pressure to be sexy goes hand in hand with the pressure to be thin, and fat women are assured that they cannot join the ranks of the desirable unless they first make themselves small. Thus the female's desires are firmly directed from a very young age toward projecting a pleasing sexual persona and away from any other form of physical gratification, so that the pleasures of food and the pleasures of sex are set up as mutually antagonistic. Food is meant to be either a marginal source of enjoyment or off limits altogether. It's as if women are expected to disavow any form of physical satisfaction other than sex, and specifically sex with men.

The woman who falls for this line of thinking and makes food her enemy thus becomes dependent upon men for what she has been taught is life's one and only legitimate physical pleasure. But a woman who enjoys food, especially "bad" foods, must worry about getting fat, and if she does gain weight, she is told that she is ugly and disturbed, and that she must choose between love and food. In fact, the biggest carrot dangled before the fat woman's nose is the lure of sexual attractiveness. If she becomes thin, she is told, she will instantly become irresistible, handsome men will flock to her, and her biggest problem will have been solved.

Could it be that a female appetite for food—a preference, even, for food over sex—represents to some people a rejection of the male as the center of the universe, a repudiation of the penis as the source of all female pleasure? Perhaps this is why a pleasure-oriented approach to food is considered neurotic, while a desire for sex for its own sake is considered healthy and desirable. After all, a heterosexual male would stand to gain many more sexual opportunities in a culture that pressures women to make sex the center of their universe to the exclusion of other pleasures. On the other hand, it's also possible that some women, married or single, who eat or overeat for pleasure do so because they are left hungry and unsatisfied by sex with their lovers or husbands.

Perhaps a large female body is threatening because on some level it represents independence, both from our anorexic cultural standards and from men as the sole givers of pleasure. Since weight bigots insist on believing that fatness is usually a conscious, defiant choice, it would follow that they would see the fat woman as a dangerous rebel with no desire to please society in general and men in particular. Conversely, perhaps the thin shape is overvalued because it represents just the opposite: an intense, even desperate, desire to please, as well as a profound dependence upon the approval of others, qualities which insecure men with weak egos would naturally find sexually appealing. And if some men are repelled by a large woman because her flesh, to them, symbolizes appetites, perhaps it is really female sexual appetites that revolt them, and they discharge that neurotic, sexist disgust by way of weight prejudice.

Food and Community: The Fat Woman Stands Alone

Finally, society's commandment that a large woman deprive herself of all "pleasure" foods raises a very basic issue: food symbolizes community. Even while our culture, like virtually every human culture, nurtures the associations between food and emotion, between eating and external stimuli, it forbids large women to participate in this relationship. We've already seen how food is wrapped up in the rituals of sex and love, but food is also a vital element of family rituals like weddings, the daily gathering around the breakfast or dinner table, and especially family-oriented "feast days" like Thanksgiving and Christmas. Then there are the social rituals—parties, holidays, anniversaries, and other special events. Likely as not, it is women who prepare and serve the food at such events, just as it is women who are instructed not to feed themselves what they are feeding others unless it is "nutritionally correct," low-fat food.

Food even plays its part in the rituals of death. In Harold Kushner's book, *When Bad Things Happen to Good People,* he describes the Jewish funeral ritual called "se'udat havra'ah," the "meal of replenishment," in which "(O)n returning from the cemetery, the mourner is not supposed to take food for himself (or to serve others). *Other people have to feed him,* symbolizing the way the community rallies around him to sustain him and to try to fill the emptiness in his world" (Kushner, 1983; italics added). Not only does Kushner's description aptly illustrate how food commingles intimately with human ceremonies, but it also shows us how society's commandment that large women eat as little as possible, and that they particularly not eat certain foods, is a powerful metaphor for its rejection of fat women as full-fledged members of the community.

To eat differently from others is to be set apart from others. In the large woman's case, she is alternately told (a) that she does not eat like thin people—i.e., she alone eats for emotional reasons and eats much more than they do—and (b) that she has no right to eat the sexual or festival foods, as they do. Dietary restrictions and differences, as with vegetarians or kosher-keeping Jews, are distinguishing markers that identify a given group of people as separate and distinct. History has shown that people who deliberately eat differently from the rest of society often arouse hostility and suspicion, so pivotal are eating habits to social identity. American society has chosen to believe that all fat people have drastically different eating habits from "normal" thin people and therefore deserve to be socially segregated.

Diet books are crammed full of sanctimonious suggestions for not "overeating"—i.e., eating any "fun" foods—at all types of social events. No matter the occasion, even if everyone around her is chugging eggnog or stuffing down the sweets, the large woman is supposed to nibble on raw vegetables or plain chicken. No doubt this accounts for the understandable resentment many dieters feel watching others engage in the culinary part of special occasions while they themselves abstain. One weight-loss writer suggests that at holiday functions you "pretend you are a diabetic vegetarian" to avoid what he calls "The Hazardous Cs—cookies, candies, cakes" (Berland, 1984b).

This same writer unwittingly acknowledges the connection between eating what everyone else is eating and full social participation when he advises the dieter, "Don't tell (your hostess) you're trying to lose weight. That is a red flag, behavior that is not acceptable during the holidays" (1984b, p. 159). And why? Because announcing a diet during the holiday season is often seen as showing off, as being above the festive and relaxed behavior at that time of year. This is just another double-bind big women often find themselves in: if they pointedly refuse rich foods at social functions, they may be perceived as self-righteous, as silently preaching to those who are partaking; but if they join everyone else at the refreshments table, they merely confirm the popular myth that they are gluttons without willpower. Damned if you do, damned if you don't. As long as she is fat, a woman is expected to stand at a distance from the rituals of love, sex, family, and even death. She is not a complete member of the social community unless she is thin, or at least in the virtuous process of becoming thin.

> *Dear Miss Manners: For a casual supper with three other couples...I baked an apple pie and took it along. I had just started a diet program and did not intend to have any myself. When my husband and I walked into the kitchen and the hostess saw my pie, she said: "Oh, you're not going to have any pie, but it's all right for the rest of us to eat it." Meaning we can gain weight, but not you.*
> Letter to "Miss Manners,"
> 1992b

Weight Prejudice in the Bedroom: The Invisible Woman as Sexual Freak

One of the most vicious elements of weight prejudice is the assertion that large women are sexually retarded and utterly alienated from their sexuality. They are told time and again that their internal sense of femininity is warped compared to the relatively normal, healthy sexuality of their thinner sisters. Some of the "thin-is-in" disciples maintain that fat women substitute food for love because they're too disturbed or unappealing to attract love, even though they want it badly; while others are sure that fat women substitute food for sex because they're afraid of sex and don't really want it at all. Still others insist that fat women engage in displacement eating either because they can't get enough sex from their lovers or husbands, or because they use fatness as an anti-sex "weapon" in their relationships to punish their mates.

> *Obese people almost always have sexual problems. The combination of grotesque fatness and repressed hostility are very destructive to closeness and good sexual relating. As anger dissipates in obese people and with it, fat, relations eventually improve.*
>
> Rubin
> *Forever Thin,* 1970

Such fragmented reasoning is inconsistent. Are women fat because they're afraid of sex or because they cannot satisfy their voracious appetite for sex? Do they eat because they want too much sex or because they want nothing to do with it?

It's no wonder, then, that some big women might be ambivalent or confused about their sexuality, considering the conflicting and uniformly negative information they receive about themselves from an early age. Why shouldn't a woman be afraid of intimacy if she is taught by bitter experience that she cannot trust people, and also that she is not perceived as female? If a young, large woman's experiences with boys and men consist primarily of being cruelly mocked or pointedly ignored, the idea of opening her emotions and her body to a class of people who readily taunt and mistreat her is quite reasonably frightening.

In her book, *Adolescence: The Farewell to Childhood,* Louise J. Kaplan, Ph.D. writes: "To become an adult the adolescent must eventually gain permission to be a person with mature genitals and reproductive capacity" (1984, p. 116). But what happens if an adolescent, primed to turn her desire and energy toward the world beyond her family, is maliciously thwarted? What if the world and/or her family refuses to acknowledge that she is a developing sexual being purely because of her size? In fact, it is a popular and vindictive myth, even among some members of the medical profession, that big women rarely become pregnant or have a healthy pregnancy/baby solely because of their weight, an opinion which constitutes the ultimate nullification of a big woman's sexuality. In such instances, is a large woman not being told that she is not "a person with...reproductive capacity"? When a fat teenager is purposely excluded from the dating scene because of her size, or when she is told again and again that she will never deserve or have love as long as she is heavy, does that not constitute a willful rejection of her as "a person with mature genitals"? Yet both these attitudes are common enough.

> As a friend of mine once told me, "Fat people make great buddies and lousy lovers."
> Richard Simmons
> *Never-Say-Diet,* 1980

Even under the most favorable circumstances, adolescence is a tricky road to negotiate, full of traps that can strand a person in some phase of social or sexual development. But when constant ridicule, humiliation, and isolation are added to the equation, puberty can become a waking nightmare of locked doors and frustration. The big teenager who finds herself in such a situation cannot go back to childhood, nor does she want to, but she may be stymied, temporarily or permanently, in her desire to go forward and participate fully in an adult world which makes clear to her that she is not welcome "as is."

Is it so surprising, then, that some fat adolescents might turn to oral gratification? Is it so unreasonable that they may consider food the only pleasure to which they will ever have access? Most likely, they will end up in the miserable yo-yo diet trap, losing weight and gaining it back, and mangling both their metabolism and self-image in the process. Thus, when society smugly points out that fat people have low self-esteem, it can comfortably pretend that all such suffering is completely self-generated and has little or nothing to do with discrimination. And when society tries to make big women believe that they prefer food to sex because they are neurotically afraid of sex, it can expediently ignore the fact that matters of sex and sexual identity are made considerably more difficult and intimidating for the large adolescent who has scorn heaped upon her for her "physically incorrect" shape.

> *The compulsive eater has an interest in being fat....the most common benefits that women saw in being large had to do with a sexual protection. In seeing herself as fat, a woman is often able to desexualize herself; the fat prevents her from considering herself as sexual.*
> Susie Orbach
> *Fat Is A Feminist Issue,* 1978

Note Orbach's peculiar choice of words—"seeing her*self* as fat," "desexualize her*self*," "fat prevents her from considering her*self* as sexual." By characterizing a large woman's sexual conflicts (if any) as primarily internal, Orbach trivializes the punitive influence of weight prejudice responsible for most, if not all, of the sexual ambivalence a large woman may feel. The good Dr. Bockar (remember the binge-and-starve diet?) also writes, "It is *we,* of course, who cannot accept our bodies, *we* who try to deny that our bodies exist...." and "...people who are fat feel bad about them*selves* and don't love them*selves*" (Bockar, 1980; italics added).

This is a common blind spot among the weight-loss preachers, one which reveals their own considerable unconscious denial. The truth is that a fat child must be taught to hate herself by the unrelenting cruelty of others, who make it plain that they hate her. A fat woman has the same capacity for sexual participation as a thin woman—but she has to be told, thousands of times and in thousands of different ways, that she is ugly and unfeminine, and she has to believe it, before she succumbs to self-disgust.

> *Why, in an era when skinny is beautiful, would a man want to make love to a woman with hips that flop about the bed like giant cushions and a belly that sags unappetizingly to her dimpled knees?... Heavy women are a drag on the dating market, and they know it.*
>
> Edelstein
> *The Woman Doctor's Diet*
> *for Women,* 1977

But weight bigots want to have a fat woman's cake and eat it, too: they must believe that her psychological suffering is entirely self-contained and self-inflicted, or else risk having to admit that they are the true source of her alienation. Thus they create a tangle of labyrinthine rationalizations to cover all contingencies. Does weight prejudice make sexual connections more difficult than necessary for many fat women? Just ask this woman who wrote into a Seattle-based sex advice column:

> *As far as I can tell, generally speaking, the following five attitudes exist in the heterosexual male community regarding fat women:*
>
> ***Perverts****: Those who think fucking fat women is just deliciously perverse. How flattering.*
> ***Bigots****: Those who believe fat women are ugly, undisciplined, etc., etc., are unwilling to acknowledge evidence to the contrary, and who rely on trashing fat women to furnish most of their Minimum Daily Pseudo He-Man Macho Confidence Requirement.*

Automatons: Those who—while not overtly abusive— have nevertheless autonomically accepted the temporarily prevailing myths regarding fat women.

Fetishers: Those obsessed with big tits/butts/thighs, but who have little or no interest in a woman's heart/mind/soul/well-being/sense of humor, etc. These may actually be decent guys and okay for a quickie, but what if one wants an honest-to-gosh relationship?

Sentients: Those straight men who are attracted to women for a variety of personal reasons that may include nuances of appearance, but which have nothing to (do) with bigoted cultural standards; who understand the marketing of hatred of fat women is up there with corsets, foot binding and other such weirdness; and who want encounters with women that are supportive, romantic, fun and sexual. I've only met men who fit into the first four categories. Do straight men who are "sentient" really exist, or was the Universe created by sadists?—One of the Healthy, Disciplined, Sexual, Sensual, Smart, Strong, Non-Overeating, Active, Pretty, Single Fat Chicks

Letter to sex columnist
"Savage Love," 1994

Unfortunately, for all its cultural lip service about sexual liberation, America is still a society with tremendous conflicts about sex and sexuality, especially female sexuality; and regardless of all the feminist discussion and rhetoric on the subject, the whore/madonna dichotomy reveals itself in full force in the stereotypes of weight prejudice. While the fat woman is occasionally assigned the "whore" role, being perceived as an example of perverse sexuality, like a freak in a circus sideshow, typically she is pigeonholed as an asexual motherly type.

Looking at ancient sculptures of fat female figures leaves one with a drastically different impression altogether, and more recent painters such as Rubens and Renoir reflect the lush eroticism and raw power of the heavy woman. But in modern America, this sensuality has been pre-empted by the anorexic shape and driven underground. Moreover, fat women are not safely hidden away by their fat, as the weight-loss fanatics contend; rather, they are perpetually battered by the condescending ignorance of a society that is forever trying to ignore, undermine or nullify their sexuality. Sometimes, though, society fails, and a breath of fresh air blows through some lucky large woman's boudoir:

> *In the five years my wife and I have been married, she has put on close to 70 pounds. Far from this being a problem, however, I discover that I love the extra flesh. My wife is 5 feet 3 inches tall and now weighs in the neighborhood of 190 pounds. We have sex every day, sometimes two or three times a day on the weekends. Now I'm wondering what it would be like to sleep with a woman who weighs, say 300 pounds or more. I'm nowhere near acting out this fantasy, but I'm wondering why I would suddenly develop this attraction to fat women, given that previously I was borderline fat-phobic and only dated slender ladies.*
>
> Letter to "Ask Isadora"
> advice column, 1992

Weight Prejudice in the Analyst's Office

In its eagerness to disown large women from the ranks of the sexual and the feminine, our anorexia-promoting culture is often illogical, but when irrational prejudice is cloaked as disinterested, rational analysis, it is perhaps at its most loathsome. Unfortunately, as we have seen in earlier chapters, portraying fat women as disturbed and pathological is not only lucrative but also provides aid, comfort, and denial to anxious and insecure "normal" people, so it's disappointing but not really surprising that the psychiatric profession would make its own contribution to sexual weight prejudice.

For instance, Marion Woodman, Jungian analyst and author of *The Owl Was a Baker's Daughter: Obesity, Anorexia Nervosa and the Repressed Feminine,* claims that the big woman's "libido is focussed on food," that she has "no understanding of positive feminine energy," and has a "fear of sexuality, spontaneous feeling, and orgasm" (1980). Although she acknowledges at the beginning of her book that "some women rejoice in their plumpness and experience no difficulties with their size" (p. 7), her relentlessly negative discussion of what she terms "obesity" virtually guarantees that no big woman, after reading this book, could even consider "rejoicing" in her size. But Woodman does not stop there. Not only does she suggest that unenlightened "obese" women face empty lives bereft of any true experience of femininity, she also insinuates that they are so physically and psychologically alienated that their own bodies may turn on them and destroy them:

> *It is significant that two of the primary cases of obesity, women who appeared healthy and totally involved in life when we did the experiment five years ago, have since died from cancer of the female organs. In both cases, the obesity was a concomitant of their inability to relate to their own femininity....The unknown demon, which possessed them for a lifetime in their obesity, ultimately showed its true face in their cancer* (p. 57).

Not only is Woodman's interpretation smug and arrogant, it is also appallingly cruel in plainly laying the blame for these women's deaths on their own failure to think psychologically correct thoughts. However, if we follow this line of reasoning to its logical conclusion, it could just as easily be argued that thousands of cases of breast or ovarian cancer among thin women are the result of their rejection of the traditional, primal feminine shape in favor of an unnatural slenderness.

Woodman's outrageous application of the concept of mind-body connection borders on the nonsensical. If one is going to ask, as she does, "What does fat symbolize?" (p. 42) as applied to women, might one not also ask, "What does shortness symbolize?" or "What does baldness symbolize?" as applied to men? It's hard to imagine any society, even ours, proceeding from the assumption that any man less than six feet tall or without a full head of hair must have fundamental, unconscious sexual conflicts. Nevertheless, Woodman states early on in her book that:

> *Two individuals may eat exactly the same number of calories and lead an equally active life. One is fat, the other thin. The fat one may, in fact, be eating less and exercising more. The essential difference lies in the individual's capacity to metabolize the caloric intake* (p. 11).

Well and good. But then she concludes, "Behind any metabolic *disturbance* there may be both physiological and psychological causes." (p. 11; italics added). In other words, even if a fat woman is neither lazy nor gluttonous, Woodman diagnoses a potentially pathological condition.

Her approach is especially hypocritical given that Jungians typically acknowledge with considerable respect the archetypal shape of femininity. Apparently, the grand and majestic form of the ancient goddess-figure is admirable as long as it remains a safe, abstract symbol; but let it manifest itself in the shape of a real woman, and fools will rush in to crush her flesh and spirit down to a more manageable size. After all, weight bigots in particular and society in general cannot afford to let women start identifying with a symbol as primeval and powerful as that of the Great Mother. They might appropriate some of that power, and they might start to throw their weight around. In her analysis of women and "obesity," Woodman has made the common but grave mistake of confusing the true hardship and suffering involved in being an object of prejudice and projection with the artificially exaggerated burden of so-called "excess" weight itself and what it supposedly represents.

Another book, *Weight, Sex & Marriage,* by therapists Richard Stuart and Barbara Jacobson, also seems to go to some lengths to accentuate the negative and eliminate the positive. The authors plainly state early on that "*over 75%* of the overweight women in our research considered their marriages to be happy" (1987). In other words, these relationships did not suffer as a result of the woman's size, as opposed to fewer than 25% who said the opposite. But did Stuart and Jacobson then go on to write a book about this majority of large, happily married women? Far from it. Perhaps reasoning that good news is no news, they write instead about the minority of big women with marital troubles based on relationship issues much deeper than post-nuptial weight gain, women whose slender bodies had failed to bring them perfect love, contentment, or personal satisfaction in the first place. Moreover, although the authors acknowledge the complicated relationship between social pressures and a woman's physical self-image, they nevertheless focus almost exclusively on the effect of a *woman's* weight in marital relations, pausing only long enough to express astonishment that heavy women with low self-esteem often find their heavy husbands as unattractive as they consider themselves to be (p. 36).

Even though it's clear that thinness is no guarantee of a fairy-tale ending in human relationships, fat women who are relatively happy are mostly ignored and invisible because it serves no one's purpose to celebrate or even acknowledge their existence. Our culture simply cannot bring itself to believe that a woman can be big *and* sexually and emotionally satisfied, or that any sexual distress related to a large body is primarily the result of America's obsession with weight, because the thin-is-good, fat-is-bad equation would then be brought into question.

> *When life is going smoothly, and weight doesn't interfere with feelings of self-worth, it's hard to find the inspiration to change. Especially when the only perceived alternative to weight gain is stringent dieting, it's easy to put off dieting*

until tomorrow—or forever—while enjoying the pleasures of today (Stuart and Jacobson, p. 12).

The fact is, many of the women presented in this book were thin to begin with and only gained weight *after* marriage. If being thin had not brought them ultimate happiness and fulfillment, why focus on weight as an issue at all? If they were married to men who either humiliated them for gaining weight or encouraged them to stay fat out of some neurotic need for control, how could weight loss be expected to help the underlying situation? Perhaps some wives who gain weight after the honeymoon are simply reacting to the shattering of that ever-popular adult fairy tale which persuades women that marriage will magically transform their lives for the better. Or perhaps some of them simply discover that, in spite of being taught that sex should be a woman's greatest source of physical pleasure, food can sometimes be just as good or even better.

As with all aspects of weight prejudice, fat women need to ask: Whose problem is it, anyway? When I overhear one woman after another verbally lash herself for not being thin or thinner; when I read one account after another of women who cringe at the sight of themselves in the mirror because their bodies are not "perfect;" and when I scan advice columns loaded with questions from young women terrified of saying "no" even to exploitative or abusive boyfriends because they are so desperate to be associated with a male, I have to wonder at the absence of strength, dignity, and self-respect which passes in this society for genuine feminine sexuality. I must consider whether the prevailing fear and hatred of fat women reflects an obsessive determination to control and destroy the formidable sexuality that a full-figured female shape has represented throughout most of human history. I am forced to ponder the denial of millennia of feminine symbolism when modern society goes to such lengths to intimidate women into making themselves as small as possible.

> *As Briffault noted again and again, among "primitive" people not yet contaminated by the physical habits and role playing of "civilization," it was common to find the women equal in stature, often larger than the men....Among Stone Age skeletons of Neanderthals it is often impossible to determine sex by size or weight of bones; early females and males were almost equal in stature, equally strong.*
>
> *As seen in the most ancient Paleolithic images of the Goddess, the solid strength and massiveness of the female body was an ideal. And certainly the human race...couldn't have survived two to three million years of catastrophic earth changes if females had been as physically weak and mentally dependent during those long, hard ages as we are supposed to be today.*
>
> Sjoo and Mor
> *The Great Cosmic Mother:*
> *Rediscovering the Religion of the*
> *Earth,* 1987

If large women are to reclaim their rightful place in society as the recognized sexual equals of thin women, they must renounce the perversely masculinized version of femininity thrust upon them. They must make it clear that they will not be bullied and browbeaten by petty tyrants who insist that the only "real" woman is one who physically resembles an adolescent with all of its connotations of malleable vulnerability and insecurity.

The big woman is equally entitled to physical and sexual nourishment. She can love and be loved; she can find just as much pleasure in intimate relationships as anyone if she is able to shake off those aspects of weight prejudice intended to smash her self-confidence and murder her libido; and she can carry life and nurture it as well as her thinner sister. She is neither sexless nor shapeless; rather, she possesses the form of the ancient and sexually formidable goddess-figures. Far from being less of a woman because of her size, she is, quite literally, more of one.

CHAPTER SIX

A Prejudice by Any Other Name

Weight Bigotry, Anti-Semitism, and the Dynamics of Discrimination

---

*In **Mein Kampf,** (Hitler) made the following comment regarding Jews: 'Their whole existence is an embodied protest against the aesthetics of the Lord's image.' Here, of course, Hitler was stating that the Jews, so hideous in appearance as to preclude their being made in God's image, were not really human....Implicit in this was the idea that what was not 'human' could not be natural.*

Robert A. Pois
*National Socialism and
the Religion of Nature*

It is a sin to be fat because that's not the way God intended man to look.

Joyce A. Bockar, M.D.
The Last Best Diet Book

The reader may ask: What is a discussion of anti-Semitism generally, and WWII-era German anti-Semitism particularly, doing in a book about weight prejudice? Three things. First, the Nazis devised and

employed a sophisticated media propaganda machine in order to in-
flame ill will toward Jews, thereby providing Germans with a
welcome scapegoat in the difficult years following Germany's defeat
in World War I. In so doing, the Nazis laid the social and moral
foundation for their very successful campaign to exclude Jews from
German society, to deprive them of jobs and of their civil rights as
citizens, to ghettoize them, to confiscate their property and thus
profit financially from anti-Semitism, and ultimately to dehumanize
Jews to the point where their very right to live could be set aside
casually and, so it seemed to the Nazis, logically.

And America? Just ask any African American about the cultural
stereotypes that relegated her people to the status of sub-human for
centuries, stereotypes employed to justify using human beings as
slaves for profit and which included a popular visual image of the
black person as an animal. Ask any gay American about the hateful
and often violent prejudice that keeps so many in the closet, or
about the images generated by homophobia of the gay person as
either a limp-wristed, lisping milquetoast or a cigar-chomping, female
thug. Ask any Jewish American who lived during the first half of this
century about exclusion from jobs, neighborhoods, and clubs, as
well as the enduring portrait of the Jew as a greasy, curly-haired,
hook-nosed villain. And ask any fat American about the mindless
stereotypes, tormenting social pressures, and discrimination which
together generate billions of dollars in profit annually for the weight-
loss industry and which cost large people so much in terms of
employment and promotions denied, unequal pay, social and sexual
isolation, alienation, and the exhaustion resulting from decades of
diets that just don't work. Ask her about the relentless imagery
characterizing fat women as diseased, neurotic gluttons and
unattractive, unlovable, second-class citizens. All prejudices, then,
involve some form of appearance-related distortion or exaggeration
that assists bigots in rationalizing their many cruelties, and weight
prejudice is no exception.

This leads us to the second reason for an analysis of anti-Semitism in this book: it is taken very seriously. Weight prejudice is such a banal and integral aspect of American culture that most people take it for granted as a natural and acceptable phenomenon. Like its targets, the prejudice itself is virtually invisible. Those who are not its direct victims conveniently fail to notice it or dismiss its significance when they do, chalk the whole thing up to mere ignorance, and advise the fat person to do likewise, not realizing that in so doing they merely exacerbate the problem. But anti-Semitism, and Nazi anti-Semitism especially, is widely considered the quintessential expression of evil in this century, and we will see in this chapter that the anti-Semite's characterization of the Jew mirrors in a number of respects the modern American perception and portrayal of the fat person. Certainly, the Nazis constructed a cultural fantasy wherein non-Nordic physical qualities reflected a degraded inferiority. American mainstream culture, for all its collective chest-thumping about rugged individualism and the value of diversity, is deeply invested in this same hollow, elitist phantasm, and fat Americans, among others, are paying the price.

The third reason for this chapter is purely personal. Growing up both large and Jewish, I had the unhappy opportunity to sample both anti-Semitism and weight prejudice on a first-hand basis for many years. I experienced too many similarities between the two prejudices to be able to ignore them. The emotions, the fundamental irrationality, and the psychological dynamics involved were basically the same; only the words used and the reactions of the adults around me were different. I also learned, too early in life, that when people require an object of hatred, they will take hold of any difference, any so-called flaw with which to flay their scapegoat. Nothing—neither facts, figures, nor appeals to humanity—will prevent them from believing what they need and want to believe. For those adults who consider anti-Semitism a serious matter but weight prejudice mere "teasing," I hope this chapter communicates how painful it is, especially for a child, to be on the receiving end of any form of prejudice, and that often the words used to inflict pain matter less than the basic cruel intent itself. Modern America is as morally bankrupt in its hysterical worship of thinness, and its attendant punishment of large women, as was Nazi Germany in its equally irrational glorification of Nordic/Aryan physical perfection.

The Patterns of Prejudice: Same Song, Different Words

In 1991, Swedish film maker Peter Cohen produced a documentary called "Architecture of Doom" about Nazi aesthetic standards and the associated dehumanization of non-Aryans. According to Cohen, the film is "about the connection between aesthetics and cruelty and violence" (Harvey, 1991). As we will see in this chapter, fat people, when they are visible at all, are typically characterized in essentially the same terms as Nazi portrayals of Jews. Nazi propaganda consistently represented Jews as fat, ugly, sloppy, dirty, and inherently unwholesome, even diseased. Now, of course, with the comfortable benefit of hindsight, we know that such concepts were the product of blind hatred, of the desperate need for a scapegoat by people who otherwise would have had no one to criticize but their government or themselves. It hardly seems a coincidence, then, that fat people are also commonly thought of as dirty, ugly, and sloppy—and as preferring themselves that way. They too are perceived by both the medical/scientific community and laypersons as innately diseased. They too serve as whipping boys and girls for a culture plagued by deep conflicts concerning food, pleasure, control, and conformity. Loudness, vulgarity, greediness, and pushiness are just a few of the qualities typically described as being peculiar to, or exaggerated in, fat people, just as anti-Semites have typically foisted these same qualities upon Jews.

The camera then pans a 'typical' Jewish home. There is a close-up of a mass of flies on a wall; the room is filthy: 'The home life of the Jews shows a marked lack of creative ability. To put it plainly, the Jewish houses are dirty and neglected.'

From *Der ewige Jude,* a Nazi
propaganda film; from
*Propaganda and the German
Cinema, 1933-1945,*
Welch, 1983

"Take P.N., 17, 157 pounds and 5'6". Color her sloppy, nervous, loudspoken, obtrusive, slovenly and lazy." (A description of a patient by a diet book author)

Schiff
*Doctor Schiff's Miracle
Weight-Loss Guide,* 1974

When a society wishes to isolate a particular group of people from the mainstream, the first step is to transform them into ugly aliens who supposedly have nothing whatever in common with "normal" people. It is no coincidence that outsider groups are identified by the single quality that distinguishes them. Hence, "the Jews." All by itself, this quality is believed to nullify whatever attributes the outsider shares with the rest of humanity, and society chooses to see only that which separates an individual from the mainstream. Accordingly, one often encounters descriptions of large people as "the obese." One diet book even goes so far as to designate big people as "overweights." Not "overweight *people*" or "overweight *men and women*"—just "overweights." How simple it becomes, then, to see a contemptible inanimate object instead of a human being.

A society bent on discriminating against a group will also artificially exaggerate any tangible difference between itself and designated outsiders; failing that, it will encourage or create a difference where one would otherwise not exist. For instance, the Nazis forced Jews to wear armbands emblazoned with the Star of

David, intending them to be emblems of shame that singled out such individuals for public ridicule befitting "subhumans." In America a fat woman, by virtue of her very shape, is often singled out for public ridicule. More significantly, attractive and fashionable clothing comparable to that available to thin women is still difficult to find and/or financially inaccessible to many large women, while others are so convinced of their own inherent ugliness and worthlessness that they would never consider buying themselves beautiful large-sized clothing. As a result, the big woman who is resigned to dark colors and ill-fitting, unflattering garments, or forced by circumstances to wear what few affordable clothes are available, will show up in public looking quite different from the thin woman who has easy access to floors and stores full of garments designed exclusively for the slender shape. Furthermore, a large woman wearing casual clothes is often disparaged as a "fat slob" while a thin woman in a sweatsuit is just that and nothing more.

It is also ironic that one genuine difference between Gentiles and Jews who "keep kosher," namely, their eating habits, is the same difference that supposedly distinguishes the thin from the fat. The observance of Jewish kosher laws (which prohibit the consumption or combination of certain foods) has long been used as an excuse to discriminate against Jews on the grounds that they are somehow dangerously different; in fact, one of the most gruesome slanders against Jews dating back to the twelfth century accused them of murdering Christian infants and using their blood to bake into Passover matzos (Scott, 1992). Likewise, fat people as a group are treated as incorrigible outsiders in the American "thin-is-in" culture because their food choices and eating habits are presumed to be grotesquely dissimilar to those of thin people. And although one diet book author after another claims that only fat people associate food with emotions, the annals of weight prejudice reveal that it is bigots who imbue food—and different eating habits, even imagined ones— with emotional, even moral, connotations.

In addition, both the Nazis and American culture have used food as an expression of power. In *The Scourge of the Swastika,* Lord Russell of Liverpool relates:

> *The (concentration) camp staff delighted in tormenting the half-starved prisoners by throwing them pieces of bread which had gone moldy in the stores. To watch these living skeletons fighting like wild beasts for such morsels was an entertainment which never failed to amuse the SS* (1954, p. 182).

To starve a person is to hold that person's life in your hands. That is power. But to persuade a person to deprive, even starve *herself* for long periods of time without ever personally withholding a morsel of food—that is supreme power, and American culture has successfully convinced millions of women that such self-deprivation is a mark of superiority and an enviable talent.

Another common tactic employed by bigots is to portray the objects of their hate as dangerously obsessed. The anti-Semite sees the Jew as a monomaniacal money-grubber, the homophobe decries the homosexual as being in a permanent and sinister state of sexual arousal, and the weight bigot insists that all fat people are single-minded gluttons perpetually preoccupied with food. For example, when, in 1993, a woman's lawsuit for weight-related employment discrimination came to the California Supreme Court, Justice Armand Arabian was quoted as saying, "If you want to eat 24 hours a day and become 305 pounds, the law doesn't give you any protection."

Moreover, this court's unanimous decision against the heavy woman aptly illustrates the indifference of American society toward righting the wrongs done to fat people. With few exceptions, employment discrimination based on weight is entirely legal in this country. How could a prejudice as entrenched as size bias have been overlooked? Age, gender, physical disability, race, religion, and creed are all qualities which receive protection under the law, but not weight, even though the practice of size discrimination is well established.

Isn't it just possible that state and federal legislators have disregarded the violation of large people's rights for decades because American culture condones the practice? Or that big people have been so effectively persuaded of their inferiority that they have been unable to muster the kind of political pull that gets results? That even people as intellectually sophisticated as state Supreme Court justices are perfectly comfortable maintaining a contemptuous and prejudicial attitude toward large people as types rather than individuals? Anti-Semitism in history has typically been underwritten by governmental and social institutions, just as weight prejudice in modern America is supported by the cultural establishment.

Another common tactic in social discrimination is to portray outsiders as taking up more than their fair share of resources, whether it be space, food, money, health care, potential mates, or jobs. A stereotype of Jews which persists even today depicts them as greedy, big-business types who hold sway over international affairs and enjoy an undue influence in the mass media. A former aide to Nation of Islam leader Louis Farrakhan described Jews in a 1994 speech as "that old hooknose, bagel-eating, lox-eating...bloodsuckers of the poor," further ranting that:

> I say you're called Goldstein, Silverstein and Rubenstein be-cause you've been stealing all the gold and silver and rubies all over the world—and it's true, because of your stealing and roguing and lying all over the face of the earth.
>
> K.A. Muhammad
> "Farrakhan, Former Aide
> Renews Attacks Against Whites,
> Jews;" San Francisco Chronicle

Fat people, likewise, are typically perceived as consuming vast amounts of food and as occupying more room than is proper; but now that health care costs have become an urgent issue in America, the heavy are also represented as self-destructive parasites whose greedy and willful self-indulgence results in an unnecessary and gross waste of medical resources. "Maybe they could charge a fat tax," one woman suggested in a news article about health habits and insurance (Fernandez, 1993). The implication here is that thin people are by comparison paragons of willpower and healthy habits, so that any waste of health-care dollars becomes a problem caused by "them."

> *Printing pieces like "Justice for the fat"...spreads misinformation and has an indirect public health effect, since it may cause some overweight individuals to be less concerned about their weight....Printing articles that play up the genetic component of obesity only makes it that much harder to convince the obese to change their lifestyles....I was especially offended by the obesity advocacy position that body weight should not be allowed to influence health insurance premiums. I strongly disagree. If I make the conscious effort to exercise and eat right, and others don't, I shouldn't have to pay for the added health care costs of those with self-inflicted higher risks.*
> Letter to the Editor
> *San Francisco Examiner,* 1994

> *Taxpayers are being burdened by these economic parasites, who get pregnant, then charge it to the taxpayers to support their follies. It is most unfair seeing these teenage mothers and able-bodied, **fat**, lazy single mothers enjoying welfare, while taxpayers work to death to support them.*
> Letter to the Editor
> *San Francisco Chronicle,*
> 1991; (emphasis added)

> *I see thousands of workers poorly dressed passing me by after a hard day's work carrying a pot of soup....They speak of their hard life and of their unbearable misery. But*

other people also pass me by clad in valuable fur coats,
with fat necks *and paunchy stomachs. These people do not*
work. They are Jews taking an evening walk....

From a speech by Julius
Streicher, editor of the Nazi-
sympathizing German
newspaper *Der Stuermer* (from
The Case Against Adolph
Eichmann, Zeiger, 1960)

Lazy Jews. Lazy fat people. "Shiftless" blacks and "wetbacks" and Indians. This pattern of bigotry is clear: the outsiders are painted as slothful leeches on society, while the insiders are the productive workers never given proper credit for their dedicated labors. Of course, the fact that society typically restricts social and economic opportunities for its manufactured pariahs is conveniently overlooked so that the latter may be comfortably condemned for their singular lack of industry and progress.

Women don't get fat because they are poor, the study (done
by Harvard) showed; they get poor because they are fat.
In the seven-year study of more than 5,000 women, the re-
searchers found that the fat women were likely to lose
socioeconomic status over the course of their adolescence
and young adulthood...no matter how well they did on
achievement tests...or whether they came from well-to-do
families.

Fraser
"The Overweight Want Their
Rights," 1994

In their book *Christians Only,* Heywood Broun and George Britt discuss an aspect of anti-Semitism which further illustrates the similarities between that prejudice and weight bigotry:

...Jews take on part of the ill-will which the rest of America
feels for New York. New York has the largest Jewish

*population, and Jewish names are associated with the
theatre, the motion picture industry, and the entertainment
world in general. And so, Puritan prejudice will vent itself
upon all and any who have a particular part in catering to
the pleasure principle* (1931, p. 15).

Likewise, "Puritan prejudice" will vent itself against fat people
because they, too, are seen as representatives of the pleasure
principle. Just as anti-Semites love to claim that Jews "own
everything"—in other words, that they have more than their fair
share of money and the personal gratification it can buy—the Health
Police are likewise convinced that the big woman is a decadent
glutton having more fun than is seemly, and so these constipated
killjoys are determined to see to it that if they themselves cannot
enjoy food, no one else will, either. For while women unconsciously
resent the cultural restrictions on their appetites, most do not dare
raise a meaningful protest for fear of the consequences, instead
finding it much safer to aim the blame at a defenseless target; hence,
the pointedly condescending animosity towards fat women, who are
popularly considered to have "let themselves go." Interestingly, this
phrase also refers to relaxed and uninhibited behavior, and in fact
it's no coincidence. So, like the Jew, the fat woman must be put in
her place and exposed for the greedy hedonist the weight bigot
wishes her to be.

Moreover, just as the Nazis demonized the Jew and
characterized Jewishness as being synonymous with every vice and
shortcoming known to humanity, so too do Americans insist on
associating fatness with drastically dangerous and destructive
habits. One letter to Ann Landers, discussing adolescent
rebelliousness, insists that "If (adolescents) want to have sex, take
drugs, drink, fail in school, *get fat,* get married, you-name-it, they will
do it" (1993c). A letter to a newspaper editor concerning an article
about the state of America's children alludes to "mounting statistics
for child suicide, violent death, *obesity,* etc." (Johnston, 1992). A
newspaper article bemoaning the loss of innocence in today's

children describes some of their artwork: "The children's crayon drawings warn against crack cocaine, teen pregnancy, *obesity,* child abuse and drinking" (Asimov, 1993). A newspaper editorial discussing AIDS education and Hispanic communities lists a series of ills suffered by the poor which includes "tuberculosis, drug-addiction, *obesity,* cancer, arthritis and dental cavities" as well as AIDS (Esquer, 1992). Yet another letter to Ann Landers about a heavy, troubled teenager brings her response that "*Overeating,* lying, stealing and cheating should not be overlooked. This is serious anti-social behavior that could lead to criminal behavior if not checked" (1993b; all italics added).

> *Inge sits in the reception room of the Jewish doctor....The*
> *Jew appears. She screams. In terror she drops the paper.*
> *Horrified she jumps up. Her eyes stare into the face of the*
> *doctor, and his face is the face of the Devil. In the middle of*
> *the Devil's face is a huge crooked nose....Around the thick*
> *lips plays a grin, "Now I have you at last, you little German*
> *girl!"....His fat fingers clutch at her. But now Inge has got*
> *hold of herself. Before the Jew can grab her she smacks his*
> *fat face with her hand....Breathlessly she runs down the*
> *stairs and escapes from the Jew's house.*
>
> Extract from a short story in a
> book for children called
> *Poisonous Fingers* (from *The*
> *Scourge of the Swastika,* Russell,
> 1954)

> *Perhaps the most memorable spot featured a smoke-filled*
> *conference room where pudgy men in dark suits discuss*
> *how 3,000 new smokers must be recruited every day to*
> *compensate for the 2,000 smokers each day who quit and*
> *the other 1,000 who die.*
>
> Lucas
> Newspaper article describing
> an anti-smoking ad, 1992

No doubt the average reader, already conditioned to see fat people as losers, at this point mentally connects every large body she sees with high-school dropouts, alcoholics, suicides, liars, cheaters, crack addicts, child abusers, violent criminals, and the like. To read these items and others like them, it is easy to see how Americans have come to believe that heavy people are not only unattractive and unhealthy, but also vaguely sinister and malevolent, potentially as great a threat to society as a drunk driver or violent drug addict. This is the same mental equation used by the Nazi propaganda machine to make Germans fear and hate Jews.

Another similarity between anti-Semitism and weight prejudice involves what psychiatrist Theodore Isaac Rubin has called "mutually exclusive superlatives," i.e., stereotypes perpetuated by bigots to rationalize their resentment and hostility towards the outsider. In the Jew's case, she is seen as:

> *Moronic, brilliant.*
> *Sadistic, masochistic.*
> *All-powerful, weakling.*
> *Cosmopolitan, provincial.*
> *Cunning, naive.*
> *Extraordinarily sensitive, calloused.*
> *Ruthlessly calculative, wildly impulsive.*
> *"Nigger-lovers," "worst bigots."*
> *Best lovers, worst lovers.*
> *Coarse and ill-mannered, polished sophisticates.*
>
> Rubin
> *Anti-Semitism: A Disease of the Mind,* 1990c

In the case of weight prejudice, we have seen in past chapters how the fat woman is perceived alternately as:

Passive, actively rebellious.

Asexual, perversely sexual.

Anti-feminine, ultra-feminine.

Denying or "stuffing" emotions, knowingly "acting out."

Childishly compulsive, maternal.
Desperate for male attention, rejecting male attention.
Disconnected from physical feelings/body awareness, yet wallowing in physical sensation with food.
Out of control, overcontrolling and domineering.

In each instance, the outsider cannot win: no matter what she does or how she presents herself, the bigot will find something neurotic in her behavior. The fat woman, like the Jew, is always wrong or sick, while the thin woman, like the non-Jew, is applauded for presumably possessing the opposite, positive qualities.

> *Lenz (a Nazi eugenics "expert") is confident that in most respects the mental powers of Nordic man exceed those of other races. He cites Fischer's observations that the mentality of the Nordic includes industry, vigorous imagination, intelligence, foresight, organizing ability, artistic capacity, individualism, a willingness to obey orders, one-sidedness,...To this Lenz adds the qualities of self-control, self-respect, respect for life and property...clarity...a love of order and of cleanliness...objectivity.*
> Proctor
> *Racial Hygiene: Medicine*
> *Under the Nazis,* 1988

> *Fat-Acceptance Groups: Collections of obese people who have banded together to convince the thin world and themselves that the things we've always known about fat people—inability to control their actions; repulsive appearance; general lack of personal responsibility; greater difficulty of movement; higher rate of absenteeism due to chronic physical problems—are, in fact, all "lies!" In other words: that the entire population of Planet Earth has been "making these things up" for the last million years or so! Good luck!*
> Rives
> *Walk Yourself Thin,* 1990

Finally, one of the more infuriating, and irrelevant, arguments promulgated by weight bigots is that since fat people have all gotten themselves into their predicament, they are not entitled to expect equitable, or even decent, treatment. Weight bigots employ this argument as a powerful lever to rationalize their prejudice. Fat people, they insist, have *chosen* to look the way they do, and therefore society's mistreatment of them is entirely reasonable. If a big person wants to stop being harassed, the thinking goes, then she should just toe the line and lose weight. As laughably oversimplified as this attitude is, it does raise a serious question: Does making an unpopular choice regarding a private matter like religion or body size justify prejudice and persecution?

The weight bigot's line of reasoning conveniently overlooks the history and foundation of anti-Semitism. Jewish people have historically paid dearly for their *choice* to remain Jewish in the face of often violent discrimination. After all, Jews could convert if they really wanted to do so. Nevertheless, non-conformity to ignorant popular standards, willful or not, is no justification for prejudice. It is pure hypocrisy for the weight bigot to condemn fat women for failing to meet society's outrageous physical standards while the bigot screams bloody murder whenever she is asked to meet the most basic moral standard of simple human decency. The issue of choice, like the issue of health, is a mask behind which the bigot can feel safe attacking her scapegoat.

A Matter of Class

*To tell the members of a group that they must move always
on tip-toe, and then only through the bypaths of life; that
they are by nature unpleasant human beings, and must
therefore never cease remaking themselves...is to ask
innocent people to behave like criminals.*
> Milton Steinberg
> *A Partisan Guide To*
> *The Jewish Problem,* 1945

"EATING TOO MUCH IS CRIMINAL"
> Inscription chiseled in stone as
> a "work of art" by Jenny Holzer
> (as reported in *Time* magazine,
> July 30, 1990)

Americans like to think that ours is an essentially classless
culture, unlike countries such as England, with conspicuous social
hierarchies. The truth is, Americans discriminate along any number
of manufactured class lines: race, religion, ethnic background,
gender, age, money, family connections, profession, level of physical
ability, sexual orientation, physical appearance generally, and height
and weight particularly. Far from being a culture blind to such
distinctions, America as a society is choked with them.

Weight prejudice actually cuts across other class lines:
perpetrators and scapegoats alike are found among men and women,
Jews and Gentiles, the young and the old, etc. In fact, while
discrimination based upon other qualities such as race or religion
may allow for positive as well as negative stereotypes, targets of
weight prejudice do not enjoy this dubious "privilege." The African-
American may be thought to have soul and sexual potency, the Jew
great intelligence and business acumen, and the Asian studiousness
and diligence, but the fat woman today gets no such credit. She is
considered altogether sad and bad inside and out, and any ideas that

she is jollier than her thin counterpart have long since fallen by the wayside.

> *Children as young as six years describe silhouettes of an obese child as "lazy," "dirty," "stupid," "ugly," "cheats," and "liars." When shown black and white drawings of a normal weight child, an obese child, and children with various handicaps, including missing hands and facial disfigurement, children and adults rate the obese child as the least likable. Not only is this prejudice relatively uniform among blacks and whites and persons from rural and urban settings, it is also, sadly, seen among obese persons themselves.*
>
> Wadden and Stunkard, 1986
> (from *Lifetime Weight Control Patient Counseling,* 3rd ed., Gustafson, 1993b)

> *Discrimination against the obese can be found in lower acceptance rates into prestigious colleges for obese high school students compared with normal-weight students, despite identical high school performances and academic qualifications or application rates to colleges.*
>
> Gustafson
> *Lifetime Weight Control Patient Counseling,* 3rd ed., 1993b

> *Much is being made about the nude 'posture photos' taken at Mills College and other elite universities from the 1940s to the 1960s, as part of a study on proving a correlation between body shape and intelligence. Pity that the research ended before photographers could drop by the NCAA Division II-level university I attended: young men with stomachs inherited from their forefathers—hearty beef-fed pouches soon to blossom into* **full-size gut sacks.** *Young women with* **Mom's cheery jowls** *and hips the width of a pickup cab. The results might not look like* **Diane Sawyer,** *but at least they would even out the curve.*
>
> Boulware
> "Slap Shots," 1995
> *San Francisco Weekly*

Another common element which weight prejudice shares with other forms of discrimination is the double standard which enables the insider group to characterize outsiders as members of an inferior class while simultaneously denying its own outrageous flaws and offenses. For example, some groups have historically made it a practice to discriminate against Jews by ghettoizing them, excluding them from certain professions, exiling them and confiscating their property, or murdering them and stealing even the skin from their bodies and the gold from their teeth, as in the concentration camps—all the while depicting the Jew as a peculiarly greedy social climber. What's wrong with this picture? Likewise, when women were sternly advised that their inborn irrationality made them incapable of practicing in traditionally male professions, men meanwhile were (and still are) picking up guns on a daily basis to maim and murder over even the smallest gesture of disrespect.

And fat people? While the diet industry hawks its mostly ineffective, often unsafe products, cynically exploiting and reinforcing cultural pressures for the sake of huge profits, it is the big woman who is portrayed as the embodiment of ravenous greed even when she is deliberately denied attendance at prestigious universities and kept away from high-paying, high-profile positions reserved for the "lean and mean."

> *Other reports note that the obese are discriminated against when they seek jobs and while on the job. Employers may rate overweight people as less desirable than normal-weight individuals, even when they think the two groups have the same abilities. In one study by Roe and Wickwort, 16 percent of employers said they would not hire obese women under any condition, and an additional 44 percent wouldn't hire them under certain circumstances. Obesity even had a dollar penalty: The researchers estimated that* **each pound of extra fat could cost an executive $1,000 a year.** *....Heavy persons are perceived as less intelligent, or as interfering or comical characters.*
>
> Gustafson
> *Lifetime Weight Control,*
> 1988a, pp. 2-13 to 2-14

While weight bigots soothe their own body-related anxieties and boost their eggshell egos at the expense of the big person's feelings and peace of mind, it is the latter who is advised that she needs to address her feelings of inferiority and anti-social hostility. And while millions of thin Americans wallow in a variety of unwholesome personal habits, it is the big person who is set apart and publicly reviled for her lack of discipline and her presumably self-destructive health habits.

In fact, the Nazis viewed women in terms remarkably similar to those of modern American culture, and their outlook mirrors not only our own obsession with rigid, narrow Nordic/Aryan aesthetic standards but also our propensity for associating body size and shape with social class:

> *All too often (Himmler's) men chose to ignore the constantly reiterated warnings against the dangers to them and their offspring involved in the choice of a non-Nordic*

woman, and the quality of the future mothers, wives, fiancees and girl friends chosen by them left much to be desired....

There were even SS men, as an officer in the SS Leithefte noted, who 'still marry short, squat girls with round figures'. According to the writer of the article, unions of this kind were undesirable for the following reasons:

1. The children would be of unpleasing (unharmonisch) appearance.

2. There could be difficulties at birth, for there was often a disproportion between the child's size and the birth passage.

3. Glandular, hormonal, disturbances are often present in such small women, particularly if they are also greatly overweight. In such cases the ability to conceive is greatly hampered, or the women are actually infertile. Also women of marriageable age who are greatly overweight are usually unattractive and in no way correspond to our Nordic idea of beauty and thus the SS ideas of selection.

> Hillel and Henry
> *Of Pure Blood,* 1976

In a survey of FAs (Fat Admirers), "17% say that having a fat spouse is a liability to one's career, 54% disagree. One respondent stated: 'I'm a blue collar worker, at my level I would have to say no. But at high level management, I would definitely say yes."

> Blickenstorfer
> "Survey of Male Fat Admirers,"
> *NAAFA Workbook*
> pp. 5-7

Likewise, the high-status Nordic woman and the high-status American woman share common physical features, as is evident in this passage from *Nazi Culture*:

> *The Nordic race is tall, long-legged, slim....The limbs, the neck, the shape of the hands and feet are vigorous and slender in appearance....The hair color is blond; among most of the existing types it can extend from a pink undertone of light blond to golden blond up to dark blond....If an illustrator, painter, or sculptor wants to represent the image of a bold, goal-determined, resolute person, or of a noble, superior, and heroic human being, man or woman, he will in most cases create an image which more or less approximates the image of the Nordic race. He will also create a man who will be regarded as a typical representative of the upper social strata* (Mosse, 1966, pp. 64-65).

In American culture, as in Nazi culture, social, sexual, and moral supremacy are assumed to proceed from conventional beauty and physical fitness; in German society, as in ours, "Images of enormous suggestive power celebrated the perfect body as the symbol of the perfect spirit" (Adam, 1992). In this description of Nazi "art" by Peter Adam from *Art of the Third Reich*, we can easily recognize the style of today's painstakingly body-sculpted models and actresses, those modern "messengers of a program imposed on life:"

> *Female sculptures were also created in abundance...of women...always full of erotic promises....The iconography was always the same: the representation of woman made by and for man....She was the fulfillment of man's desire. But the study of these women reveals nothing natural. What dominates is a forced body style, artificial poses, and affected eroticism* (1992, p. 188).

*Everything about them (the sculptures **The Army** and **The Party**) is idealized: their hair, lips, bodies....Everything is noble, even the material, and yet they look hollow and totally artificial.*

The National Socialist figures strike a pose....How could people have thought that these figures represented real persons, real living beings?....Breker's statues are cold and self-contained. In short, they radiate a superbly tailored lifeless perfection. These statues are merely the messengers of a program imposed on life (p. 200).

Adam's words illuminate the choice forced upon every outsider in relation to social mobility and the standards of so-called perfection set purposely beyond her reach. Should she get with the "program" and strive for a "superbly tailored lifeless perfection?" Does she accept society's curse upon her, that by her very existence she offends even God, or does she search for meaning beyond an oppressive class system? An observation by Milton Steinberg in *A Partisan Guide To The Jewish Problem* illustrates the dilemma equally applicable to the Jew and the fat woman: "On how far the Jew must go in remaking himself there is little agreement. Some feel that he need eliminate only external and flagrant differences; others demand that he recast his very soul" (1945, p. 70). The ultimate question, of course, is: whose soul is it, anyway?

In *Anti-Semite and Jew,* Jean-Paul Sartre terms anti-Semitism "a poor man's snobbery...propagated mainly among the middle classes, because they possess neither land nor house nor castle, having only some ready cash and a few securities in the bank" (1948, p. 26). Weight prejudice functions in a similar fashion. Rare indeed is the thin woman who actually leads a life which reflects the popular fantasy of perfect love, health, and success; and vilifying heavy people provides the former, no matter how poor, lonely, or ignorant she may be, with an unquestionable cache of superiority. She can always relieve her own feelings of frustration or inferiority by sneering at the "fat girl," no matter how wealthy, well-loved, or accomplished the latter might be. Likewise, the heavy woman battered by bigotry may play "kick the cat," in turn passing judgment on anyone heavier than she: I may be bad, she will reason, but at least I'm not as bad as you. Hence, the condescending ridicule of large ladies even when they make it to the top of their profession. No matter how good a person the big woman is, no matter how successful she becomes, her weight will be treated as a mark against her, so that she is still subordinate to the thinnest lout in the land.

In one respect, American social regimentation is more sinister than overt and blatant prejudice such as that found in Nazi Germany because it masquerades as a benign influence. It sugarcoats the pressures exerted by disguising them as a wholesome concern for health or as a casual and harmless personal preference. But whereas the Nazis also considered good health to be a "moral, one might almost say a legal obligation" (as noted in a Nazi handbook for training the Hitler youth), they made no pretense of embracing individualism, while American culture devotes large amounts of lip service to the glorification of diversity and equal opportunities for "the pursuit of happiness." However, judging from the fairly constant level of modern social protest, our popular culture seems to alienate far more people than it supports, so apparently there is a sizable discrepancy between the ideal and the reality. In any event, Americans are not tolerant of visible differences, and physical appearance is considered a significant marker of class distinction. As one scientist doing research on the effect of looks upon social standing flatly stated, "Appearance is so important to our opinions of other people, it's almost disgusting....Attractive individuals, adult or child, are always preferred" (Blum, 1992).

At Arm's Length: Prejudice and Segregation

A good way to tell if a particular group suffers from the slings and arrows of bigotry is if its members are somehow segregated. European Jews, of course, were often forced to live in walled ghettos which were locked up each night to keep them away from their "betters." In America, Jews had to fight for the right to live in the same middle-or upper-class neighborhoods as Gentiles as well as for access to decent jobs and fair pay, facing formidable opposition to their efforts to achieve social and economic equality. Anti-Semites, meanwhile, did their best to keep Jews segregated in a ghetto without walls, surely a familiar situation to many fat people in America today.

Social isolation is a convenient tool for bigots of any kind who are interested in maintaining the status quo. As long as the bigot can keep the outsider literally and figuratively outside and out of sight, there can be no uncomfortable challenges to carefully tended stereotypes. In a magazine survey about fat people, the remarks of one slender teenage girl aptly illustrate this vicious game of "keep-away:"

> I really feel for those who have trouble with their weight, but if you were with a bunch of your friends, and they all started to laugh and call someone names because they were fat, you wouldn't tell them to stop. You would do it also. I have been in this situation many times and, yes, I called them names. I also felt guilty afterward. I don't think many of us would invite a person who is obese to our party or to spend the night, much less be friends with him or her. I really don't think I would.
>
> Elkus
> "What it feels like to be fat,"
> Minton, 1992

> Using Jews as alien people and outsiders provides the anti-Semite a synthetic source of belonging....This reinforce-

*ment of identification with the national majority becomes
necessary during attacks of inadequacy and eruptions of
dependency feelings. Being an "insider" gives synthetic
strength that is fed by isolating the Jew in the crowd,
separating him from the crowd and viewing him as
"outside."*

*The long-standing and habitual process of depersonalizing
and dehumanizing Jews (part of the process of separating
them from the whole and sustaining their alienation)
makes it easier to deaden what shades of conscience and
moral equivocation might still exist in the anti-Semite.*
                              Hillel and Henry
                              Of Pure Blood, 1976

One place where both Jews and fat women have had occasion to
find themselves unwelcome is the swimming pool. In *Anti-Semite and
Jew,* Sartre noted that "The first thing the Germans did was to forbid
Jews access to swimming pools; it seemed to them that if the body of
an Israelite were to plunge into that confined body of water, the
water would be completely befouled" (1948, p. 34). In America as
well, certain neighborhoods, hotels, and country clubs—and their
pools—were once off-limits to both Jews and African-Americans.

Now, while big people are technically free to visit the local
beach, pool, or gym if they so choose, they are also quite likely to
encounter some degree of hostility to their presence:

*I'm fairly tolerant of bodily variations and imperfections,
such as Cindy Crawford's (a famous model) mole, but it
really bothers me, aesthetically, to walk along the beach
and see so many guys with overhanging guts and plushly
upholstered "love handles." I can live with fat thighs, up to
a point. I'm not real keen on the zaftig zeppelins who
apparently intrigued Rubens and Renoir.*
                              Carey
                              "Losing weight for bathing-suit
                              season," 1993

Magnanimous as this gentleman thinks he is, a great many people are not nearly so generous, and they are more than eager to express with great energy and volume their displeasure at seeing an exposed body that is not taut and thin. As a result, some large women now organize separate swim and exercise classes to avoid such discouraging and prejudiced treatment, creating a self-imposed segregation.

The fat person, like the Jew, is also familiar with the quiet sort of segregation in the workplace that involves keeping her away from fast-track jobs. According to one NAAFA survey,

> *Over 40% of fat men and 60% of fat women stated that they had not been hired for a job in the past because of their weight. In contrast, almost none of the non-fat respondents indicated that this had ever occurred. Over 30% of fat men and women indicated that they had been denied promotions or raises, and over 25% indicated that they had been denied benefits (such as health or life insurance) because of their weight. Nearly 70% of fat men and women had been questioned about their weight on the job or urged to lose weight, and this was also true of about 30% of moderately fat people and 10% of non-fat people.*
> *NAAFA Workbook,* pp. 6-13

Of course, a big woman's qualifications for a job mean nothing if an employer believes the myths of weight prejudice, myths once applied vigorously in the case of American Jews:

*One of the most thorough studies of the causes of employment discrimination against Jews was made by Bruno Lasker, and published in the **Jewish Social Service Quarterly** of March, 1926. This was based upon direct questions to employers who advertised that they would not take Jews. Among the replies were the following:*

"Our past experience has proved that Jews and Gentiles do not work together very well, and the former we never found remarkable for cleanliness, etc."

Broun and Britt
Christians Only, 1931

Sound familiar? Compare the above with these two statements regarding fat people on the job:

*If I have two equally qualified (people) for employment, one **thin and well-dressed,** the other **obese and dirty**...if I follow this ordinance (an appearance-oriented anti-discrimination ordinance passed in Santa Cruz, California) I have to discriminate against the **thin, clean** one or I go to court.*

Ratner, "Santa Cruz Gives
Tentative OK To Law on
Personal Appearance," 1992;
(emphasis added)

Absenteeism, poor job performance, low productivity, depressed morale—these are just some of the potential consequences of having overweight employees.

1992 letter sent out by
Weight Watchers to employers
advertising their At Work
program

Furthermore, heavy women are precluded from engaging in occupations whose prerequisites include extreme weight restrictions, just as Jews were once restricted in their choice of profession. If you travel by air you are unlikely to encounter a flight attendant who is even slightly heavy, and members of the military may face discipline or discharge if they exceed a certain number of pounds. Columnist Anna Quindlen, writing in 1993 about airline weight limits for flight attendants, noted one such attendant who wore a size 10 dress and weighed 144 pounds, yet faced a threat to her career if she did not get down to 135 pounds. Another attendant was suspended without pay for being twelve pounds "overweight" at 145 pounds. Also in 1993, a naval petty officer with four good-conduct medals was threatened with a dishonorable discharge, also for being twelve pounds over the Navy's weight limits. The big woman may even be restricted from occupying certain front-office positions for which she is qualified, thanks to a preoccupation with a slick and sleek corporate image or a macho "harem" mentality which considers a workplace with high-visibility "babes" a reflection of a male boss's superior status and potency.

In sum, the big woman, like the Jew in both Europe and America through most of history, is set apart. She must shop separately from thin women, read separate magazines if she wishes to see herself fairly represented, go to separate social events if she wants to be recognized as a normal human being, and keep on the lookout for special TV shows that speak to her and her situation. Even when she occupies space in the same classroom, office, store, neighborhood, sometimes even the same bedroom, as the thin person, the big woman is on some level considered a "special case," an alien relegated to what amounts to an alternate universe. Plainly, this is not the manner in which a society treats its first-class citizens.

"Blondes Run the World"

One reason for this inequitable state of affairs is that while Americans comfortably condemn German Nazis for goose-stepping into line with the barbaric values of the Third Reich and its notions of racial purity, we nevertheless actively support an outlook that parallels the aesthetic and ideological foundations of Aryan supremacy. American culture would not put such a premium on tall, slender, blue-eyed blondes, nor endow them with such an exaggerated aura of glamour and status if it were not deeply enthralled by the Aryan myth of superiority based on looks. If Americans were truly disgusted with the fascist aesthetic-moral philosophy—that people with Nordic physical qualities are more valuable than those who are different—then we would have discarded, or at least minimized, such standards long ago. This is not the case.

Although this book is not about the vices or virtues of blondness, this chapter is concerned with the similarities between two cultures which both succumbed—happily enough, it would seem—to a powerfully materialistic and alienating cult of the body. For the Nazis, a blonde head attached to a perfect form held a much deeper significance than just an attractive sight, and America has also embraced this attitude with gusto, so that today thinness, like blondness, has acquired a powerful symbolic meaning which goes far beyond the physical characteristic itself. Likewise, the fat woman has assumed the same role as counterpoint to the slender blonde in American social mythology as the stereotypically short, squat, dark-haired, hook-nosed Jew played to the Nordic warrior in Nazi Germany. In fact, those short, fat brunettes referred to by Lois Wyse at the beginning of this book who are not "allowed to enter California" are undoubtably classified as outsiders partly because they bear such a strong resemblance to the American stereotype of the European Jewish peasant woman.

Consequently, female celebrities with Nordic features, like Marilyn Monroe (thin in her time, not in ours), Meryl Streep, Michelle Pfeiffer, Kim Basinger, Melanie Griffith, Darryl Hannah, and Sharon Stone, to name just a few, are viewed as exemplifying glamour and style, combining sexual charisma with class. According to one study after another regarding appearance and status, "Psychologists have found that attractive people are widely regarded as being more intelligent, friendly, honest and confident than others" (Marshall, 1993). In *Blonde Beautiful Blonde,* Ms. Wyse quotes, quite correctly, that "...blonde hair, blue eyes, and white teeth are still the American media's—specifically television's—most marketable commodities" (1980, p. 37).

Nazi propagandists, like American media moguls, also manipulated the media very shrewdly to reinforce a social hierarchy expedient to the ruling class; and as Peter Adam has pointed out in *Art of the Third Reich,* "The evil in the National Socialist regime lay in the fact that, as Hannah Arendt observed, it decided who had the right to live. And art was used to drive this message home" (1992, p. 110). A similar message is driven home by the American mass media which, as we have seen, fiercely promotes and sustains the myth of the slender blonde superwoman to considerable commercial and social advantage. And while Nazi culture has provided a powerful historical lesson on the inhumanity of any substantive connection between physical appearance and social/moral worth, our own culture shows not the least interest in learning this lesson.

> *Of course it takes more than blonde hair to make a blonde appealing. It also takes a blonde body. The **best** blondes are in shape and shapely, and exercise keeps them looking fit (Lois Wyse; emphasis added).*

All my life I've felt better, special because I'm blonde. (Cathi Black)

Blondes live, think and act better than brunettes....Blondes run the world. (Sally Jessy Raphael)
Lois Wyse
Blonde Beautiful Blonde, 1980

Certainly, inane remarks like these reveal a deep-seated engagement with the concept that a certain kind of "look" implies a clear superiority. If we could transport the multitudes who worship at the altar of the slender, blonde sex symbol back in time to 1930's Nazi Germany, would they reject the irrational myth of Aryan superiority? Given the pressures to conform—pressures much harsher than in our culture today—would they be offended by the notion that buff Nordic types are better, more beautiful, more entitled, more exciting and dynamic? It's an ugly but reasonable question, and likely the answer would be even uglier.

Of course, women of color don't typically come with blue eyes and golden hair, so the cult of the thin blonde contains a strong thread of racism as well. Likewise, the implication that "in shape and shapely" women are the "best" is just as elitist and arrogant as the insinuation that only blonde—and presumably white—women "make the grade."

In conclusion, let's compare Ms. Wyse's—and America's—blind worship of the California girl type with this quote from a former inmate of the World War II concentration camp Auschwitz who had the misfortune to come in close contact with one of The Beautiful People. Notice how the former prisoner makes special, careful mention of the Nazi's physical appearance, almost as if she herself could not comprehend the behavior of one so attractive:

I knew an S.S. Arbeitsdienstfuhrer Hasse at Auschwitz. I would describe her as about 28 years of age, about 5 ft. 8 ins. in height, very blond hair (natural), straight, and worn in an upward style, blue eyes, blonde eyebrows, small mouth, round face, healthy complexion, slim build, good even teeth, beautiful, good figure, and very smart in her dress.

This woman was in charge of the transport columns which arrived at Auschwitz from time to time....She used to lead the columns to the gas chamber, and where there were babies in arms, she ordered them to be thrown into a hole which was connected to a stove, and they were burnt alive. I was employed in cleaning up the ground near the crematorium and I saw this happen many times.

Statement of Helena Kopper
(Hungarian, aged 35)
Zeiger
*The Case Against Adolph
Eichmann,* 1960

The best blondes, indeed.

Back to the Future: Eugenics and the Unfit, Then and Now

Historians exploring the origins of the Nazi destruction of lives not worth living have only in recent years begun to stress the links between the destruction of the handicapped and mentally ill, on the one hand, and the Jews, on the other. And yet the two programs were linked in both theory and practice. One of the key ideological elements was the "medicalization of anti-Semitism"—the view developed by Nazi physicians that the Jews were "a diseased race," and

that the Jewish question might be solved by "medical means."
> Robert Proctor
> *Racial Hygiene: Medicine Under the Nazis,* 1988

We have already seen in earlier chapters how "excess" weight is popularly viewed as an automatic indicator of physical and psychological disease. We have also seen how the "medicalization" of weight prejudice, like that of anti-Semitism, serves as a mask for pervasive social and economic discrimination. What we will see here is that American proposals for solving the "obesity question" have a good deal in common, ideologically speaking, with the pseudoscientific Nazi consideration of the "Jewish question." Like Europe's Jews, big people in America are officially designated as society's "unfit."

Nazi physicians also claimed...that Jews actually suffered from a higher incidence of certain metabolic and mental diseases....Interesting as well, Wagner noted, was the fact that Jews showed a higher rate of sexual deficiency, expressed, for example, in the blurring of secondary sexual characteristics....Wagner concluded that Jews were "a diseased race;" Judaism was "disease incarnate."
> Robert Proctor
> *Racial Hygiene: Medicine Under The Nazis,* 1988

*Obese people almost always have sexual problems;... obesity is **sickness**—an emotional sickness or neurotic state of mind, call it what you will **but** understand that the obese man or woman is **sick**.*
> Rubin
> *Forever Thin,* 1970a

Certainly, the American scientific/medical establishment seems never to rest in its quest to "fix" fat people. Dieting is still heavily promoted, despite its proven inadequacies; nevertheless, even though medical science is finally beginning to wake up to the futility and long-term ill-effects of this weight-loss method, it still refuses to acknowledge that human beings naturally come in a variety of sizes. Instead, drugs and surgery appear to be the up-and-coming treatments of choice. Finally, there is the burgeoning threat of genetic discrimination combined with the potential for genetic engineering. Whatever the approach, the big person is made to understand that she, like the Jew, is biologically and/or psychologically defective; she is persuaded that she must override her genetic programming by any means possible if she is to achieve normalcy.

It's also important to keep in mind that there were many perfectly qualified German scientists and physicians who eagerly researched and developed "evidence" of Jewish physical and mental degradation and inferiority, and their collaboration with the Fascist anti-Semitic crusade should convince us once and for all that science, far from being an arena of pristine objectivity, can be twisted and manipulated to create conclusions that collude with popular prejudice.

The Nazis used such pseudoscientific evidence as a flimsy justification for condemning millions of people to exile, imprisonment, torture, and death, although these decisions were sometimes based solely upon an individual's shape, size, facial features, eye and hair color.

*Persons were also selected for execution from those detained in hospital. I have seen the patients made to run naked past the selectors and those who could not run quickly or looked ill or poorly developed or, **in the case of women, were ugly,** were picked out by any of the selectors present.*

> Zeiger
> *The Case Against Adolf Eichmann,* 1960; (emphasis added)

While fat women are not systematically executed for their weight, they can and do face a peril to their physical well-being when doctors consciously or unconsciously set a separate and inferior standard of care for their heavy patients. Decades of yo-yo dieting, stress, isolation, weight-loss drugs, and surgery also pose a threat to the big woman's survival.

Even the federal government now seems ready and willing to participate in this intrusive agenda. On December 6, 1994, first Lady Hillary Clinton and former Surgeon General C. Everett Koop launched "a campaign to get people out of the refrigerator and off their backsides." Called "Shape Up America," the campaign coincided with the release of a report by the National Academy of Science Institute of Medicine on weight loss, a report which "analyzes and evaluates various ways of dealing with obesity, including diets, exercise, *appetite-suppressing drugs and surgery*" ("The Slimming of America," 1994; italics added). Apparently, the Institute believes that "Anti-obesity medications and surgery, for example, 'deserve a new look as potentially powerful and effective weight-management treatments, if used properly, for some people,' specifically those who have failed with other approaches...." Of course, since the failure rate for diets is generally placed at 75-90%, this would provide the medical profession a wide berth to prescribe expensive drugs and even more expensive surgery, none of which have yet been proven to be either safe or effective.

Amazingly, the Institute of Medicine scientists suggest that re-defining obesity "not as a cosmetic problem but as 'an important, chronic, degenerative disease'" will contribute to "a growing move-ment to promote more tolerance toward those who are overweight and an increasing body of scientific evidence indicating that obesity probably has metabolic and genetic underpinnings" (Cimons, 1994). What they conveniently overlook is that fat people are already defined as inherently diseased and pathological, and that such an attitude has done absolutely nothing to "promote tolerance," and everything to promote weight prejudice. The Nazis defined Jewishness as a moral, psychological, and physical disease; did that "promote tolerance" toward Jews? Quite the contrary.

Finally, the Institute of Medicine report suggests that weight-loss medication be administered on a long-term basis rather than several months' duration. And yet a 1994 article in the *Wall Street Journal* proposed that "Safety and Long-Term Effectiveness of Diet Drugs Are Still Uncertain," citing short- and long-term side effects such as "short-term memory loss, headache, diarrhea and nausea," and further stating that "studies don't offer reassurance that the drugs are safe to prescribe as medication for the rest of a patient's life" (Miller, 1994).

The antidepressant Prozac, for example, is under consideration as a weight-loss drug; however, the dosage prescribed for slimming purposes is reportedly triple the dose prescribed for depression (Miller, 1994). Apparently, Prozac does not magically make the pounds melt away; it simply causes a loss of appetite, or anorexia, as noted in the *Physicians' Desk Reference* entry for Prozac. Do doctors consider a long-term loss of appetite a desirable condition? The underlying assumption here appears to be that the big person's eating patterns are typically so drastically out of control that those appetites which cannot be "fixed" by willpower or regular diets must be decimated by drugs.

In addition, the *PDR* reveals that "in controlled clinical trials, ap-proximately 9% of patients treated with Prozac experienced anorexia" (p. 944), a percentage which hardly seems to justify the use of such a powerful and controversial drug. On the contrary, under "Adverse Reactions," the listing acknowledges frequent *increased* appetite and infrequent weight *gain* (p. 946). Some of the other common side effects of a normal Prozac dosage include "nervous system complaints, including anxiety, nervousness, and insomnia; drowsiness and fatigue or asthenia [physical weakness]; tremor; sweating; gastrointestinal complaints, including...nausea and diarrhea; and dizziness or lightheadedness" (p. 945). Chills, abnormal dreams, agitation, and bronchitis are also listed as frequent adverse reactions (p. 946). Whereas risking such side effects may be worthwhile when Prozac provides relief from a serious disease like depression, the idea of using it on a long-term basis purely to induce anorexia simply illustrates the medical establishment's poor priorities and indifference to a more meaningful definition of health for fat people which emphasizes good nutrition and physical activity, without regard for weight loss.

Of course, if Prozac is not approved as a weight-loss drug, there's always the old standby, PPA (phenylpropanolamine hydrocholoride), which can be purchased without a prescription in diet pills such as Accutrim and Dexatrim. As long ago as 1983, the authors of *Over The Counter Pills That Don't Work* expressed concerns about this weight-loss drug which was "originally marketed as a nasal decongestant:"

> *Despite the (FDA) panel's decision (rating PPA safe and effective), it is our opinion that PPA poses a substantial hazard for its users, and has not succeeded in proving its effectiveness.*

Not only are there significant questions of PPA's effectiveness, but also serious doubts of its safety. PPA can cause hypertension (high blood pressure), even in young, healthy adults given amounts within the recommended dosage.

There have been cases of potentially fatal heart problems, kidney disease and muscle damage associated with the use of (PPA)-containing products....There have also been reports of amphetamine ("speed")-like adverse reactions to PPA-containing products. These include accelerated pulse rate, tremor, restlessness, agitation, anxiety, dizziness and hallucinations. These reactions may be aggravated by the presence of caffeine in many of these products (Kaufman, et al., 1983).

In early 1995, CBS' "Eye to Eye" did an update on this drug. The PPA industry, predictably enough, insists that the drug is safe, but according to one doctor interviewed on the program, "It is possible to have severe, life-threatening reactions such as stroke or heart attack after just taking one diet pill." Furthermore, this doctor "personally knows of 30 cases of strokes directly linked to PPA." The update went on to say that:

There are other studies linking PPA to paranoid psychosis, cardiovascular problems, and stroke, so four years ago the National Institutes of Health funded a study which found 142 instances of severe problems associated with the drug, including 24 brain hemorrhages and 8 deaths....It may surprise you to know that after two decades on the market and scores of studies, PPA still has not gotten final approval from the FDA. That's because these pills were being sold long before the FDA began regulating over-the-counter drugs. They were presumed to be safe, and still are.

It certainly is a Brave New World for the fat person. A 1991 news article even speculated on the possibility of someday synthesizing a protozoan parasite capable of preventing fat absorption in the human digestive system. The article indicates that "It's not clear if pharmaceutical companies have begun to explore this parasite's potential—but there's no question that such research would be both technically feasible and possibly enormously profitable" (Schrage, 1991). Would it be cynical to suggest that some doctors and pharmaceutical companies are currently looking for a significant piece of the financial action that weight-loss programs and over-the-counter diet pills have so long enjoyed? Indeed, the *Wall Street Journal* article quoted earlier indicates that "the drug industry is placing some big bets that the market for obesity is ready to explode," and also, incidentally, that a year's prescription for Prozac runs $600 to $1,400 (Miller, M., p. A6).

If these and other weight-loss medications under consideration fail to prove themselves as magic bullets, there's always the last-ditch resort of surgery to "fix" the big person: liposuction for slightly to moderately fat people, and stomach stapling and the like for extremely heavy people. According to *The New Our Bodies, Ourselves*:

> *Even worse than dieting are the various types of surgery medicine offers women labeled obese. They include carving fat off, jaw wiring and various ways to make the stomach and intestines smaller, decreasing a person's ability to eat and thereby absorb nutrients. These operations are performed almost entirely on women, may have a death rate as high as 10 percent and are only moderately effective in achieving the stated goal of weight loss....After intestinal tract operations a woman often gets severe diarrhea for several months and is at higher risk of getting gallstones and arthritis, two problems supposedly 'cured' by weight loss* (Boston Women's Health Collective, 1984, p. 22).

One man and his mother who both underwent stomach stapling experienced such extreme side effects that the "disease" of obesity must have been heaven compared with the misery inflicted by its "cure." Between the two of them, they endured severe pain and bloating, cramping and severe vomiting, rapid weight loss, dizzy spells, weakness, a calcium deficiency, loss of teeth, hair loss, bone problems, hernias, a stomach ulcer, electrolyte and potassium deficiencies, and heart problems, followed by depression (Jablonski, "The Cutting Edge," 1993). Another woman who submitted to stomach stapling suffered from intestinal gangrene, abdominal infection, and kidney failure before dying 17 days after her operation (*NAAFA Newsletter,* 1992). One surgery patient who had her stomach stapled in 1979 and lived to tell about the ensuing physical and emotional horrors wrote, "Am I lucky to be a weight loss *survivor?* The lucky ones have already died" (Eckert, 1992). Far from sounding like a miracle "cure," weight-loss surgery and its consequences conjure up mental images of gruesome medieval tortures—or of Nazi medical experimentation on Jews and other expendable, "unfit" concentration camp prisoners.

On the other hand, while the medical profession seems to be straining at the bit for the chance to prescribe dubious weight-loss drugs and surgery, some of its members may at the same time be reluctant to provide big people with life-saving medical treatment. Dr. Dean Edell has written that doctors deciding who is eligible for an organ transplant will sometimes "deny someone an organ that could save his or her life" purely on the basis of the patient's weight, simply because obesity is considered a surgical risk. He goes on to say that:

> *...obese patients had proportionally about the same number of complications and blood clots as the leaner group, and spent about the same amount of time in the hospital recovering. Most important, obese patients weren't*

any more likely to reject their organs, and their survival rate after three years was just as high" (Edell, 1992).

Could it be that, like the Nazi physicians who considered the lives of the mentally or physically disabled "not worth living," some American doctors function under the assumption that the lives of the unfit—i.e., fat people—are similarly unworthy of medical resources?

> *To make a long story short...Candy had a brain aneurysm, which sent her to the hospital for emergency surgery. When she had a second surgery a week later, the doctor indicated that the first surgeon had botched up the job, with stitches slipping and bone fragments left in. It wouldn't surprise me if the first surgeon let things slide, let Candy down, because he didn't think she was worth it, because she was fat.*
>
> Smith
> "In Memoriam"
> *NAAFA Newsletter,* 1992

> *Dr. John Redelfs lost his medical license in June (1991) after a patient went into psychotic withdrawal from amphetamine-like drugs he prescribed for her to lose weight. But because the 70-year-old doctor shredded his patient records, authorities now say they can't tell whether he complied with a court-ordered plan to protect other patients who may be in danger....He (the doctor) balked at contacting several hundred (patient) because he couldn't afford the cost....'I do not feel guilty,' he said....After a lengthy investigation, state medical authorities found that Denise L. (the psychotic patient) had been taking amphetamine-like drugs under Redelfs' supervision for nearly seven years....*
>
> Bailey
> "Shredded Records Muddle
> Doctor Case," 1991

As if all this weren't enough, the invisible and "unfit" woman has still more to look forward to from the priests of high technology. Genetic research is making great strides in identifying the DNA markers for all sorts of diseases. According to Dr. Paul Billings, chief of genetic medicine at the California Pacific Medical Center, "The FBI is collecting genetic information....The insurance industry has large computer banks. The army is collecting a DNA sample from every recruit. This will soon back up the largest genetic data bank in the world." He reminds us as well that "until World War II and the horrors of the Nazi Holocaust, 20 U.S. states had laws allowing the forced sterilization of 'imbeciles,' alcoholics and other 'mental defectives;'" also, that "The sterilization law in California was the model for one of the racial hygiene laws in Nazi Germany" (Lattin, 1992). Meanwhile, the French government recently decided to introduce legislation that:

> *...will seek to prevent parents from selecting or determining physical and mental characteristics of the future child....French officials said the government is particularly alarmed by advances in medical technology that now made it feasible for women to choose the ethnic identity,* **physical size** *and other characteristics of their baby through embryo implants."*
> Drozdiak
> "France May Ban Test-Tube
> Babies For Older Women," 1994;
> (emphasis added)

Knowing as we do how the average scientist or physician, as well as the average American, feels about even moderate "overweight," this bit of technological so-called progress begs the question: will future embryos be designed to generate only perfectly slender individuals? Will American genetic technology someday achieve what Nazi genetic scientists only dreamed of doing? And what would such "breakthroughs" mean for the quality of life of large people already born?

> *...the revolution in genetic medicine turns out to have a dark side as well: Insurance companies and employers already are using genetic tests to deny health care coverage to healthy individuals who are at risk for developing a disease years later....Dr. Paul Billings, chief of genetic medicine at the California Pacific Medical Center in San Francisco...documented 93 cases of "genetic discrimination" in which insurers and employers made decisions to limit or deny health care coverage based on the results of genetic tests.*
>
> Barnum
> "Insurers Use Genes to Deny
> Coverage," 1992

> *German physicians recognized that the presentation of detailed medical records (to determine a person's genetic 'fitness' to marry and reproduce) before a court without the permission of the patient altered the traditional privacy of the doctor-patient relationship; medical journals in the early years of the Third Reich frequently discussed how the rights of individuals to have their medical records kept confidential appeared to conflict with the broader obligation to maintain the genetic health of the German population. The question of privacy was ultimately resolved by requiring physicians to report cases of genetic illness in the same way they were required to report births and deaths or certain infectious or venereal diseases, and so forth.*
>
> Proctor
> *Racial Hygiene: Medicine Under*
> *the Nazis,* 1988

If the Nazis were capable, without so much as a flicker of conscience, of sterilizing or murdering children so that they could not reproduce "inferior" individuals, of enslaving and slaughtering millions of what they termed "subhumans" to stabilize and reinforce their world-view of the Nordic individual's superiority, what then are Americans not ultimately capable of if the national obsession with physical appearance as a measure of human worth continues to escalate? Is it stretching things too far to think that if amniocentesis were to reveal a fetus with the mere *potential* for obesity, that fetus might be aborted because of the parents' fear that the child would suffer discrimination, or, worse, because of the parents' own distaste for a baby that was less than "perfect"? How far are Americans willing to carry their love affair with "good" looks, and what price are they willing to force supposedly unfit, unattractive individuals to pay for their failure or refusal to conform? Will it stop with social injustice and employment and health-care discrimination, or will the pressures grow more intense? Will heavy women continue to be invisible in the influential mirror-world of the mass media, or will they eventually be "eliminated" with questionable "wonder" weight-loss drugs and/or surgery, so-called solutions which are now apparently sanctioned by the federal government? How deep and how long does the American public need to wallow in its anorexic, flesh-free fantasy of absolute, rigid control over women's bodies?

In her book, *Perfect Women,* Colette Dowling writes of a "deadly defensiveness that consumes anorexics operating in many perfection-seeking women," of "bodybuilders who have little sense of joy in their bodies, but are motivated by the same 'emphasis on will, purity and perfection' that drives women with eating disorders" (1988). To the extent that America has taken the philosophy of aesthetic fascism to heart, it, too, is joyless, parched, and consumed. The American obsession with physical perfection, like the Nazi infatuation with the idea of a "pure" race, has nothing to do with joy or even striving for one's personal best, but is really a wild-goose chase after the vacuum of invulnerability—which is often all that the illusion of perfection truly represents. Every punitive caste system is fueled by a craven terror of inadequacy and the attendant psychological exposure, and weight prejudice is no exception. The fat woman, like the Jew, is conscripted by society to carry its collective burdens of self-hatred and fear; how else could she possibly inspire the giddy heights of self-satisfaction one sees so often in weight bigots as they concoct one pathetic rationalization after another for their many cruelties? The fat woman, like the Jew, is visible to cowards and bullies only as a type, never an individual; and the fat woman, like the Jew, is never good enough no matter what, simply because bigots do not wish, indeed cannot bear, to see her as an authentic human being.

> *He hath disgraced me, and hind'red me half a million, laughed at my losses, mocked at my gains, scorned my nation, thwarted my bargains, cooled my friends, heated mine enemies—and what's his reason? I am a Jew. Hath not a Jew eyes? Hath not a Jew hands, organs, dimensions, senses, affections, passions?—fed with the same food, hurt with the same weapons, subject to the same diseases, healed by the same means, warmed and cooled by the same winter and summer as a Christian is? If you prick us, do we not bleed? If you tickle us, do we not laugh? If you poison us, do we not die? And if you wrong us, shall we not revenge? If we are like you in the rest, we will resemble you in that....The villainy you teach me I will execute, and it shall go hard but I will better the instruction.*
> Shakespeare
> *The Merchant of Venice*

CHAPTER SEVEN

Invisible No More

Learning to be Seen and Heard

---

*I hate a song that makes you think that you're not any good. I hate a song that makes you think you're just born to lose. Bound to lose. No good to nobody. No good for nothin'. 'Cause you're either too old or too young, or too fat or too thin, or too ugly or too this or too that. Songs that run you down, songs that poke fun at you on account of your bad luck or your hard traveling. I am out to fight those kinds of songs with my very last breath of air and my last drop of blood. I am out to sing songs that prove to you that this is **your** world.*

Woody Guthrie
Bound For Glory

As we've seen, the American landscape is littered with all kinds of "songs" meant to persuade the fat woman that she's not any good— "born to lose, bound to lose, no good to nobody, and no good for nothin'." She is faced by constant challenges to her individuality, femininity, and humanity. She would be pardoned for wondering if this really is her world. In *The Beauty Myth*, Naomi Wolf recalls Simone de Beauvoir's observation that no man is truly free to love a fat woman. "If that is true," Wolf writes, "how free are men?" (1991) Likewise, no woman in America today is at liberty to be even slightly fat, so how free are women?

It would be marvelous if the big woman could wake up tomorrow to a life without so many unnecessary obstacles between herself and love, happiness, success, and a sense of belonging. For now, though, she is stuck with a culture that masquerades as expansive and individualistic even while it conveys the message that there is only room enough in this country for one size of woman, and the smallest size at that. She must still face a world that views her with contempt and makes little or no effort to disguise it. She must still cope with a society which callously rejects her yet also tries to keep her dancing at the end of its strings by demanding that she exhaust herself trying to gain social approval. And if she raises her voice to protest the constraints which weight prejudice places upon her will and ability to live well, she must still contend with angry people who, denied their traditional scapegoats by "political correctness," aim to keep her on at all costs as the last whipping girl they can flay with impunity.

All this leaves the big woman with a dilemma: since she cannot ignore this world except at her peril, how can she best negotiate its poisonous tricks and traps? Should she grant the thin world the benefit of the doubt, she who is so often denied it? Should she adopt a "live and let live" attitude which insists that, while beauty and health come in all shapes and sizes, at the same time beauty and health are not acceptable criteria by which to measure human worth? Or should she try to displace the anorexic shape with her own, and take every opportunity to express disgust for thinness as the essence of pinched, parched, anal-retentive ugliness? Should she act as an agent of the saying, "What goes around, comes around"? The big woman's freedom must begin with an understanding of the political and ideological ramifications of the common, everyday pressures and expectations surrounding her. But where does she go from there?

Is Beauty the Beast?

The popular social practice of using beauty as a means of measuring a woman's worth has taken quite a beating in recent years, and with good reason. Beauty is a real beast when it becomes a religion unto itself, complete with cynical disciples and the worship of hollow, narcissistic values. Beauty is supremely ugly when having it becomes so important that a woman feels paralyzed, or is dismissed as worthless, without it. But must the big woman wholly reject the very concept of beauty in order to reclaim some dignity and pleasure for herself?

No. While it's undeniable that current standards have grown far too narrow and inflexible, beauty is a beast that can be tamed, but only if women stand up to it. It is imperative to give modern notions of beauty a makeover, as it were, so that it is incidental, rather than central, to a woman's identity, and to expand the definition of feminine beauty to include more women—real women—rather than excluding the majority and thus burdening them with the suffocating frustrations of a manufactured inferiority. We must remember that there is a world of difference between stating on the one hand that a thin woman can be beautiful, dynamic, interesting, etc., and on the other that *only* a thin woman can possess such qualities.

On the subject of female beauty generally, there is often a failure to recognize any middle ground, which, although neither especially dramatic nor sensational, could provide the breathing room American women require. While I consider myself a tough-minded feminist with a zero tolerance for sexism, I nevertheless enjoy elegant clothes, jewelry, perfume, etc. I enjoy the admiration and company of mature men of all ages who don't think of women as toys, trophies, dolls, or dogs. It's been my experience that most women also enjoy some or all of these things.

At the same time, I have very strict limits to what I'll do, buy, or believe to achieve anyone's version of beauty. Some years, beauty rituals seem like a monumental waste of time, money and energy, and I'll have nothing to do with them; other times, I find them enjoyable and entertaining, and I indulge myself to the hilt—to please myself and no one else. Alternating between one phase and the other, I've learned that feminine sexuality is a powerful and impersonal force of nature which endures quite nicely with or without manicures, perms, makeup, or society's imprimatur.

As for weight, I was thirty years old when at last I took a hammer to my scale (which never gave me a consistent reading in its nasty, short and brutish life). I knew then I had reached the point of no return. I knew that whatever my physical appearance, I would never waste another moment waiting for permission to feel feminine, eat good food, or enjoy my body in its supposedly "imperfect" state, because I finally realized that in a culture as obsessively controlling, materialistic, and immature as ours, such permission would never be forthcoming.

Accordingly, *what* a woman does to achieve a sense of beauty sometimes matters less than *why* she does it. If she participates in the more harmless beauty rituals for her own enjoyment, she need not feel anxious or apologize for herself. However, if these become dreary duties which she resents, weapons which she cynically deploys against those whom she perceives as her enemies and competitors in a feminine rat race, or if she fears being less of a woman, less valuable, without all the accessories—in short, if being conventionally pretty constitutes the very foundation of her identity, that's when the red alert should go off in her mind. Likewise, when a woman takes risks with her health, emotional well-being, even her life, just to be beautiful, she has stepped over the boundaries.

Ideally, beauty rituals should amplify the femininity every woman already possesses and feed her natural sensuality—not constitute femininity itself. They should be pleasurable experiences free of anxiety, pain, or risk, rather than instruments of an adolescent, elitist social hierarchy. They should serve the woman, not the other way around.

After all, how many men would wear steel corsets around their torsos resulting in breathlessness, frequent fainting, and pressure on their internal organs—just to be thought handsome? How many men would periodically starve themselves, eating only tiny green salads and acres of rice cakes—just to look more attractive? How many men would treat their own bodies as a fearsome and hated enemy? Women, on the other hand, have historically mutilated themselves and their daughters (and pressured others to follow suit) in any number of ways because they are carefully and deliberately persuaded that their survival and access to love and/or social status depend upon it.

Moreover, women are typically the emotional glue in human relationships. Society exploits this situation by promoting empathy and emotional vulnerability as properly "feminine" qualities, thus carefully training women from a young age to respond viscerally to the needs and opinions of others, a process which renders women psychologically suggestible. It is a simple task, then, to tame even the most outspoken rebel by threatening her with wholesale abandonment by the community. Gaining weight? Better watch it; no one loves a fat woman. Can't lose weight? Better buy this, or you're doomed to spend your life poor, friendless, and alone. This is the trap in which so many women find themselves ensnared, strictly socialized to care endlessly about the likes and dislikes of family, friends, and even total strangers. The American woman's obsession with weight and her willingness to base her entire worth on her measurements is a neon sign blaring her low social rank. Clearly, when beauty does behave like a beast, and a woman lets it back her into a corner, she's bound to end up in a cage herself.

Blaming the Victim

One thing women should *not* do: blame the victim. What is blaming the victim? It's suggesting that a person who gets upset or angry about weight prejudice has low self-esteem. For example, a former co-worker of mine, a large woman, heard about this book through a mutual acquaintance and reportedly suggested that it was too bad that I had "bought into the fat-girl" stereotype, as if by protesting prejudice I was somehow reinforcing it.

Blaming the victim also means achieving personal happiness and then forgetting all about the other big people in the world, especially the big children, who have little or no moral or emotional support and who are still suffering and struggling for some simple dignity. It's saying, or implying, "I got mine, and if you don't have yours, it must be all your own fault. Just change your attitude, and everything will be all right."

For example, in 1993, when *Ladies' Home Journal* editor Leslie Lampert wrote about the constant abuse and discrimination she encountered while wearing a "fat suit" constructed to make her look quite heavy, *BBW* magazine's Janey Milstead replied to those experiences in article of her own. Milstead suggested that since she herself, a proud and confident fat woman, rarely faced the kind of daily bigotry which Lampert described, it was probably Lampert's own discomfort and self-consciousness that "attracted" the ridicule. What never seems to get mentioned in this sort of dialogue, however, is the fact that thin women are not required to muster self-confidence just to make it down the street, walk into a restaurant, or ride public transportation without being casually humiliated. Even if a thin woman is swamped in self-loathing and depression, she need not endure being stared, snickered, or jeered at as long as she blends into the crowd. Rather, it is the big woman who must never let herself appear to be sad, ill, or tired lest the predatory weight bigot pick her out of the crowd as vulnerable prey.

176 THE INVISIBLE WOMAN

Moreover, if we apply the "asking for it" philosophy to other forms of prejudice, we can see the hollowness of such reasoning. When the African-American loan applicant is turned down because of her skin color, is it her fault for not exuding enough self-respect? When a woman takes a position in a predominantly male profession and is faced with sexual harassment, is it her responsibility for harboring internal self-doubts? When a gay person is verbally or physically attacked for her sexual orientation, is it because she was "projecting" personal confusion about her self-worth? This type of thinking teeters dangerously close to the suspicions which so many rape victims must endure after being attacked: what did you do to encourage this? What could you have done to prevent it? You must have a "victim" mentality, or it wouldn't have happened.

It is one thing to maintain that big women should develop emotional strength so that when they do encounter prejudice it does not blindside them; it is quite another thing to insinuate that big women "attract" prejudice because they're not wearing sufficiently pretty clothes or because they're not relentlessly cheerful. Unfortunately, while the comfortable and the content want only to believe that all is right with the world and that the misfortunes of others are somehow magically deserved, it is ultimately the uncomfortable and the discontented who are forced to point out the injustices which others cannot or will not see. Big women need to realize that weight prejudice is a systemic social problem rather than a byproduct of their own personal failures; otherwise, they will continue to blame themselves for the thin world's expedient misjudgments.

In fact, the growing number of industries and associations (such as NAAFA) for the large-sized, including magazines like *Big Beautiful Woman* and *Radiance,* would never have gotten off the ground or enjoyed even moderate success had there not been a problem in the first place, if weight obsession had not driven big women into an impossibly tight corner with nowhere to go. This is not to say that developing a good self-image is not of the utmost importance in dealing with bigotry. At the same time, though, low self-esteem neither justifies nor explains the harassment and discrimination which many big women must face. Just as it is weight prejudice, not weight, that is the source of so much pain, it is the insecurities and inadequacies of the weight bigot, not her scapegoat, that are at the root of the trouble.

Furthermore, telling a fat woman that the best way to fight weight prejudice is simply to ignore it is no better philosophically or psychologically, and no more effective, than telling her to lose weight and fit in. When I was very young and tormented almost daily by other children for my size, my parents quite coolly told me, "They're just ignorant. You'll just have to ignore it." What they meant was, "It's not our problem, so don't bother us with your messy emotional needs." As a result, I grew up thinking that the endless taunting was all my fault, that something in addition to being fat was wrong with me since, try as I might, I could not manage to let it all slide off my back. Not only was I a failure physically, but also emotionally and psychologically. No one, of course, ever suggested that the failure lay with the weight bigots in my world; no, the flaw was entirely mine for "letting" it happen by being fat to begin with, and also for letting it bother me.

Some big women who have had the good fortune to be exposed to relatively little weight prejudice promote the attitude that weight bigotry doesn't matter, that the prejudice is insignificant and should be treated as such. Not only is this wishful thinking, but it reflects an inability to empathize, a failing which is unfortunately not restricted to bigots. But if you are a heavy child or youth for whom every day among your peers is a living hell of humiliation, weight prejudice matters. If you are a heavy woman who is deprived of a job opportunity for which you are well qualified because the employer is a weight bigot, it matters. If you go to a doctor who sees nothing but your weight and treats—or mistreats—you accordingly, and your insurance permits little or no doctor-shopping, it matters. If you are forced to pay extra premiums for your health insurance, or are unable to obtain coverage at all purely because of your weight and regardless of good health habits, it matters. If you are excluded from the local social and sexual scene purely because of your weight, it matters. If you are discriminated against in the workplace because of your weight and attempt to obtain justice by way of litigation, you will find out very quickly in most states that high self-esteem and good health habits are entirely irrelevant in a court of law. Weight prejudice is *not* a one-on-one problem that can be fixed by saying, "I like myself, so it doesn't matter." It does matter.

Nevertheless, people who believe prejudice can be dispelled by a show of dignity are sure that bigots will see the error of their ways if faced with big women who exude self-respect. This depends largely on a prejudiced person's level of emotional dependency upon popular stereotypes. If weight prejudice is only a casual assumption to which she has given little or no thought, then the odds are better that she can be induced to rethink her position. But if someone has a substantial emotional investment in perceiving heavy people as ugly, lazy, unhealthy, etc., and if giving up that perception means admitting a serious mistake and raising these supposedly inferior people to her own level, then it is less likely she will surrender her expedient, self-serving stereotypes, regardless of proof to the contrary.

A hardcore bigot usually has serious personal problems of her own, and the loss of scapegoats to so-called "political correctness" deprives her of an indispensable distraction from her own flaws and misfortunes. What this means for the heavy woman is that in many cases she is derided as ugly even if she dresses elegantly, moves gracefully, and has classically flawless features; she is called sloppy no matter how much time and effort she puts into personal grooming; she is considered lazy and unlovable even if she has a meaningful career and a happy family; and she is assumed to be neurotic and self-indulgent regardless of how comparable her eating habits are to those of many thin women.

An Eye for an Eye

Is the solution, then, for the fat woman to take all the self-hatred dumped on her and dump it right back onto the thin woman? To inflict countless humiliations and then treat her victim's ensuing anguish as a casual joke or a conversation piece—even as an opportunity to make money? An eye for an eye, etc.?

No. It is impossible to hate with impunity, even when the hatred is justified. Whenever we actively seek to exclude, when we behave as if someone else is, as Woody Guthrie said, "no good to nobody" or "no good for nothin'" just because of her size, age, religion, etc., we are responsible for the pain we cause. Whenever we contribute, in however small a manner, to the suffering of others, telling them they are not "real" women or men because of the way they look, we awaken and nourish rage. This is why I included the last part of Shakespeare's "If you prick us, do we not bleed?" Shylock speech in an earlier chapter.

> *And if you wrong us, shall we not revenge? If we are like you in the rest, we will resemble you in that....The villainy you teach me I will execute, and it shall go hard but I will better the instruction.*

This is the ultimate, long-term danger of scapegoating: not only does it dehumanize both victim and tormentor, but it can inspire a terrible hatred and hunger for vengeance. I know from personal experience how powerfully tempting it can be to reciprocate the high-handed cruelty which the world dishes out to fat people so liberally. I long for the day when I can finally forget the leering faces of my cowardly childhood tormentors who waited for the pain to show on my face, like vultures waiting for a death rattle. But there are inevitable consequences for using and abusing innocent people in the name of beauty, health, and corporate greed; and thin women will have to swallow some cruelly bitter medicine should the big woman ever regain the favored status she once enjoyed in times past.

And yet, the everyday heroes around us and the heroes of history are those who have declined to avenge suffering with more of the same. Christ, Gandhi, King—they all refused to return pain for pain, teaching us that power-mongers work to emphasize differences, to divide and conquer, while visionaries unite people and show us how much we have in common. This is supreme courage, the greatest human strength: to break the chain, to refuse to grant one's tormentors the flattery of imitating them. For the innocent individual who has been viciously ridiculed day after day, year after year, it may also be the most difficult course to choose.

But every outsider, sooner or later, is forced to face the moral question: do I want to be part of the problem or part of the solution? Do I wield my rage and frustration like a club, lashing and battering anyone outside my own group? Or do I acknowledge my anger and then deliberately set it aside? Do I represent "my" people as perfect martyrs who can do no wrong, who are above all criticism and completely beyond reproach, or do I recognize that no group has a monopoly on either good or evil? Do I help to unite, or to divide?

Unfortunately, the all-or-nothing quality of the thin-is-in credo precludes the possibility of genuine communication. If a big woman considers everyone thinner than herself an enemy or competitor, she cannot see the price the thin woman may pay for her status and opportunities; e.g., being treated like a trophy, getting lost in a shallow, meaningless life of narcissism, or always having to wonder if she is loved for her looks or herself. Likewise, as long as a thin woman is preoccupied with conforming to the anorexic norm, she cannot see that a woman can be large and authentically feminine, and can live a good life in spite of weight prejudice. When such blindness is mutual, women of all sizes remain imprisoned in a feverish mental maze of pressures, expectations, inadequacy, and competition. Is this freedom?

The Fruits of Liberty

Nevertheless, many people still equate perfection, especially physical perfection, with freedom—freedom from criticism, from ridicule, even from loneliness or the obligation to treat others decently. What if women could be persuaded that this wasn't true? Why bother trying to be perfect if it's not the solution to every problem or sorrow? Why crave the attention of those who can only care for you if it's the easy and fashionable thing to do? Losing weight purely to appease bigots is like a Jew converting just to please anti-Semites, or a black person bleaching her skin in order to try and satisfy racist tastes. It's like eating in the shadow of the millions of busybody weight bigots who expect every large woman to lead a docile, meager life full of anxious measuring, so that with each bite of food she takes, a woman involuntarily calculates society's approval or disapproval. It is, in short, emotional slavery.

On the other hand, releasing yourself from the petty—or should one say petite?—tyranny of calorie- and portion-counting and yo-yo dieting is a supremely liberating experience. Imagine giving yourself permission to eat anything you want, whenever and wherever you want, and as much as you want, without struggling mentally or feeling guilty. Imagine intentionally detaching all moral content from the acts of eating and exercising. Eventually the automatic anxiety and self-reproach fade away, and your relationship with food becomes more relaxed. You and you alone are in complete control of your body. You find better things to do besides worrying about food and avoiding (or being preoccupied with) mirror images. You begin to regain the energy that has been drained by self-hatred and unrealistic expectations.

You may even discover, if you choose to try, that exercise can be exhilarating when you do it because it feels good instead of dragging yourself to it because it's something you have to do to lose weight.

Maybe your weight goes down. Maybe it goes up. Maybe it stays the same. So what? This is your life now.

When you reach beyond the demands, expectations, and pressures of others to find your own needs and desires, diet and exercise issues gradually untangle themselves from issues of power, pain, and conformity; they no longer determine whether you are good or bad, worthy or unworthy, inferior or superior. Freedom means not wasting time, money, and energy trying to live someone else's idea of a good life. Whatever choices you make, you are in charge, and that is a feeling worth more than all the perky weight-loss ads and loose clothes in the universe. You are eating for one person now, and one person alone: yourself. You are free.

Women With Nothing to Prove: No More Apologies

In an earlier chapter, I quoted Shulamith Firestone, who wrote about the "exclusivity of the beauty ideal" and how women who refuse to play the beauty game risk the loss of their "social legitimacy" (p. 152). The early suffragettes risked a great deal more than this so that later generations of women could have the vote and other basic democratic rights. When English suffragettes staged protest fasts in prison, their jailers would hold them down and force-feed them by ramming a plastic tube down their throats or up their noses into their stomachs—a potent illustration of the use of food as power (Adam, R., 1975). We should also bear in mind that the feminists of past generations lived in a much more restrictive culture than ours today. But they fought and they risked, and the rest of us are reaping the benefits.

What about us? American women are under constant pressure to establish and maintain our social and sexual authenticity by means of our measurements first and our personalities and accomplishments last. If we are to reclaim our dignity and our bodies from those who insist on seeing women as babes for the using and the taking, competition to be kept down, or walking, talking jokes, then we must be willing to make some changes.

At the very least, we must stop talking about our bodies as if they were our enemies. We must stop whining about how much we hate ourselves because we don't wear a size 4 or 6, thereby communicating to one and all that self-respect begins and ends with a "perfect" figure. We must stop hanging our heads at each snide remark and every harping advertisement or commercial or billboard or movie or personals ad hammering into our heads the idea that being thin slender fit trim slim petite svelte willowy lean fragile is a woman's only hope and salvation. We must stop snickering and sneering at each other for being anything else. We must renounce the social hierarchy that places thin women on the top of the social heap at the expense of large women, and we must discourage the social inertia that shrugs off injustice just because it is the familiar status quo. We must, in the words of Carole Shaw, founder and former editor of *Big Beautiful Woman* magazine, STOP APOLOGIZING for ourselves.

Fortunately, some women are at last beginning to question the rights of others to judge them on the basis of their dress size. More large people are finally developing the perspective and the courage to look weight prejudice in the face, see it for what it really is, and come through the experience with their self-respect intact. The following are two conversations I had with big women who have wrestled long and hard with this issue, women who, while not unaffected by weight prejudice, have a solid understanding of what it is and how it is used to control women.

Mary and Sophia

Mary (all first names have been changed) is a divorced working woman who's currently in a relationship with a man who finds her shapely the way she is and has no interest in changing her, which is fortunate because Mary displays neither the intention nor the desire to conform to society's outrageous physical standards. She speaks in a very no-nonsense sort of way, and conveys a strong-minded sense of independence. She also refuses to submit to other people's ignorance and their expectations that she keep to life's sidelines.

Sophia works as a massage therapist. She is single and has a teenage son. Although she possesses the gentle acceptance of others one often finds in people in her profession, Sophia is also adamant about living life her way and on her own terms. Like Mary, she adapts her eating and exercise habits purely to suit herself and her own internal needs, rather than someone else's idea of how she should look. She believes women should learn to like themselves as they are, and especially hates to hear big women berating themselves about their weight.

Sophia: [to Mary] It takes a hell of a lot of self-esteem. You put yourself out there, on the line. You're not letting those attitudes [about your weight] stop you from getting what you want, which is someone to share your life with.

Mary: Well, I think I'm a healthy person. That's what has gotten me out there in the dating game, because I know I'm healthy. That doesn't mean there aren't days when I'm sad or feeling inadequate in some way because of my weight, but for people whose self-esteem is very low, I think part of the problem is that they don't get out there to be with people. I've actually made four or five male friends; we agreed we weren't interested in each other for a romantic relationship but liked each other anyway.

The relationship I'm in right now is with a man who's very physically fit, very active. I would say we balance each other out because he knows that I'm trying very hard to be more active, although not focused on dieting. When I first met him I said, "Look, I'm not losing any weight for anybody; either you like me the way I am or not at all. Now that you've met me, and you seem to like me, I want you to take three or four days to think about this. If you still think you want to see me, and my weight's not an issue for you, and you're not thinking about changing me, then call me." And he said, "I don't need time to do that." He doesn't ever say, "You've got to lose weight," or "I don't feel comfortable with you." I don't feel like he's trying to change me; I think he's just accepted me for who I am. I think part of why John sees me as he does is that he doesn't live his life for his friends.

WCG: *So he doesn't have this peer group that's pressuring him to have a perfect babe that he feels he has to show off in front of them.*

Mary: *Right. I think that's good in the sense that he's an independent type, and society isn't controlling him. Whether I lose weight or not has nothing to do with anybody else, not even with him. It's really all about me.*

WCG: *So you're more interested in being active and feeling good than in fulfilling some little size 6 fantasy.*

Sophia: *I think we all have to get to a point in our lives where we really live for ourselves. I'm not going to allow society to dictate to me what they consider "overweight" or "underweight," what looks good to them or what looks bad to them. I've resolved for myself what looks good to me and what's comfortable for me, and it may not to you or anyone else, but to me it does.*

Mary: *Did you see the paper today? There was an article saying that if you're a woman who's 5 feet tall, you should weigh 100 lbs., and for every inch of height, add 5 lbs., so I should weigh 115 pounds. Baloney! I will never be 115 pounds, I don't want to be 115 pounds, I refuse to be. I will be whatever I want to be. It might be 150 pounds, it might be 140 lbs. If I feel healthy, and I'm still as active as I am today, that's it. I dance a lot, I cycle during the summer for 40 miles at a time, and my weight does not limit me. My focus is on healthy eating, not losing weight for society.*

WCG: *I think it was Virginia Woolf who said that every woman should have a room of her own. You can take that literally or on a psychological and emotional level as well. Every woman should have a room of her own in her mind where she can decide what's right for her even if everyone around her is saying, "I'm not going to like you unless you become what I want you to be." But it sounds like you've worked out a way to get around that kind of pressure so you can decide what you want rather than letting all these little voices saying, "Fatandugly, fatandugly" determine what you're going to do with your body and your life.*

Mary: *If I had allowed society to do that to me, I wouldn't be dating at all. I've lived a life with a lot of pain in it for a lot of years, but what life's really about now is that I want happiness and I'm not going to let anything get in my way.*

WCG: *When it comes to food, would you consider yourself a compulsive eater? Because that's the automatic label that people will slap on you; if you're not a size 6, you must be a compulsive eater who's thinking about food all the time.*

Mary: No. I would say I have my days when I look at food as
        something that's very nurturing; I have my days when I
        just feel hungry, and I have days when I don't really care
        about eating at all. But I don't sit down and eat an entire
        bag of chips at one sitting, I don't lock myself up in a
        room and gorge all day; that's not the kind of person I
        am. I'm pretty much a person who eats three meals a
        day.

WCG: [to Sophia] You must have some interesting stories since
        you're a massage therapist and you work with women's
        bodies all the time.

Sophia: I constantly deal with this. I hear women—mostly
        women—talking about how fat they are, how overweight,
        how horrible they look, just constantly, and I'm fed up
        with hearing women talk about themselves like that. It's
        really forced me to look at myself and my body, who I
        am, what I am, and what I want for myself.

        When I was at my heaviest, 195 pounds, my male clients
        would come in with a "Hey, buddy, hey, pal" type of
        attitude towards me, just a real friendly kind of
        relationship. Or else they would come in and ask all
        kinds of questions about Susan, the tall blonde....

WCG: The tall, **thin** blonde.

Sophia: Uh-huh. Now, of course, she thinks she's really fat,
        because she's put on a couple of pounds, and she thinks
        she's grotesque. It's horrible! I think a woman is much
        more desirable, much more beautiful, when she's heavy.
        I honestly believe that.

        These men would come in and they would be asking
        questions about Susan and about other women there, and
        they would talk to me as their friend. And that would be

all right, because as a massage therapist I have very strong boundaries, and I don't let male clients know anything about my personal life. But now that I've lost weight, almost every male client who comes through the door will say something like, "Sophia, you know you really look great," and they look right at my waist and my breasts.

Mary: And they're not looking at your face.

Sophia: It makes me sick. I went to my goddaughter's baptism this Sunday, and a lot of the people there hadn't seen me for years, and I was disgusted with these people. All night long it was, "Sophia, you look great, "Sophia, I've never seen you look so good," "Sophia, I didn't recognize you," "Sophia, I can't believe it's you," "Sophia, look at you!" "Sophia, you look fantastic," "How did you do this?" "Oh my God, how much weight have you lost?" A few times I even said to some of them, "You know, I didn't know that I looked so damn bad before. Excuse me!" It really devalued me as a human being. I said to them, "Think about what you're saying." Other people are much friendlier to me since I've lost weight.

WCG: It's as if that's the central issue by which they judge you.

Sophia: Absolutely. As soon as clients that haven't come in for five or six months see me, that's the first thing that comes out of their mouths. To me, that's really sad.

WCG: You've said that a lot of women won't come in for massages because they don't feel thin enough to get undressed around a stranger, or that they don't feel they're worth it because they're not thin. And even when they do come in, they're embarrassed.

Sophia: Absolutely. They feel like they have to excuse themselves for being heavy, and it's even more so now than it was when I was heavier. They didn't feel so uncomfortable then. I can sense it right away. I let them know that I recently lost weight and that it wasn't for "the look." I truly do not judge people by their bodies; I don't do that. It angers me when people devalue themselves because they're heavy.

I have a male friend who's always telling me, "Honey, what the hell do you want to lose weight for?" It is so refreshing to hear a man who appreciates larger-sized women for what they are. He says he loves lying next to a woman in bed and really feeling the roundness, softness, and warmth of a large body. He said he was with a thin, big-breasted woman once and it was a big turn-off for him physically. She was very pretty, but he likes big women.

Mary: I'm still self-conscious about my body, but my boyfriend is perfectly okay with it. He lets me know that he's not judging my body, that he's attracted to shapely women. He touches my body and tells me that I am shapely, in such a way that my body doesn't feel so cut off and uncomfortable. I believe that my ex-husband always judged me for my weight. I remember one night shortly before the marriage ended, when we had another couple over for dinner. I cooked a nice meal, and excused myself for a moment and left the room. Upon returning, I overheard the other man say to my husband, "You can do better than that. You're a good-looking guy, and she's just a fat bitch."

Louise

Louise is married with two young children and works as a hairdresser. She grew up as the only heavy person in a family with six children, an alcoholic mother preoccupied with thinness, and a father for whom she could never lose enough weight. She has been surrounded since childhood by the message that thin is good and fat is bad, but she has never put her life on hold because of her size. An extremely friendly woman with a great sense of humor and equanimity, Louise is determined not to pass on to her children the destructive lessons about weight and personal worth she learned at home.

Louise: I've got five brothers and sisters, and they're all thin except me; I've always had to struggle with my weight and they always let me know it. I think they're obsessed with weight, and I feel less loved because I'm "overweight." It's kind of sad.

WCG: But your husband doesn't do that, does he? He loves you any which way.

Louise: Yes. He always makes me feel attractive, whatever my weight. I never notice a difference. The way he touches me, his kindness, it's always the same, whether I've gained or lost weight. He's really great. I could have on clothes that are too small for me, and he'll say, "Looks nice." He won't say anything about it. He's struggled with his weight, too.

I remember one time when I was seven months pregnant and we drove three hours to see my parents, and the first thing my father said was, "I want to talk to you." So he says, "I think you need to lose weight, and I think your husband needs to lose weight, too." I said, "I'm seven months pregnant, and who cares what you think about *my husband?" I also pointed out to him that he'd been a smoker for a long time, and if and when people make a change, they do it when they're ready to do it, not because someone's harping at them. But it was the first thing out of his mouth after we drove three hours to see them—that I needed to go on a diet.*

WCG: *It sounds like a real power play. Is that what your parents do with food and weight issues?*

Louise: *Oh, yeah. It's a way to make you feel guilty, and they do it with other things, too.*

WCG: *Have they been doing that all your life?*

Louise: *Yes. I can remember being younger and struggling with my weight and my mother saying things like, "You don't need any more, you've had enough!"*

I try to be very aware of these issues with my two children, because I don't want them becoming anorexic or having other eating problems. I never, ever try to force them to finish everything on their plates, I just let them eat until they're full. Actually, they're very good eaters. They eat their three squares and they have healthy snacks, and they're not real big on sweets. I do keep some sweets around because it wasn't around when I was growing up. My mom's always been a big health nut—she's an alcoholic, too—it's really odd, she's an alcoholic and she walks some 15 miles a day. Anyway, I try to keep everything around so my kids can try everything so they won't be obsessed or feel deprived. I don't push anything on them.

I was out with my mom for lunch one time and she was telling my son, "If you finish your lunch, I'll buy you an ice cream cone." Well, I'd ordered a hot dog for him, and it was really big and he was only three at the time, but he ate almost the entire thing except for a couple of bites. My mother said, "I'm not going to buy you that ice cream cone unless you finish that lunch." My son was saying, "But I'm full, I'm full." I said, "You know, Mom, you're not the only person with a dollar." I told my son he could have an ice cream cone later if he wanted one and he didn't have to finish the hot dog. But it really made me aware of how my mother plays that power game with food.

I could be in the grocery store with her and she'll see someone who's really heavy and she'll say, "Look at that. Look at that." And the person's right there, and I tell her, "I don't want to hear it. Just be quiet." I'm afraid the other person's going to hear it, and I know how it feels when someone makes a comment about my weight. But you can't tell my mom anything about her problems, because she's pretty much perfect as far as she's concerned.

WCG: *Has your five-year-old son ever expressed a sense of shame about your size?*

Louise: *No. He's always been really good about complimenting me. He'll come in and say, "Oh, Mommy, that looks so nice on you," or "You look so pretty." If I buy new clothes and model them for the family, he'll stop playing and say, "Oh, Mommy, that's so pretty," and my husband will look up over his newspaper and say, "Oh, yeah, that looks nice."*

WCG: *Have you thought about how you'll talk about weight when your two-year-old daughter gets older?*

Louise: *Oh, yes. One of my customers was planning to go on a trip to visit friends, only she told me she didn't want to go because the woman friend she'd be visiting had lost a lot of weight, so my customer didn't want to go because she was heavy and this other woman had lost weight. So she said, "Oh my God, we can't go!" And her little girl was saying, "Why can't we go?" And the woman stopped herself, and then said, "We're going." She realized that she didn't want to do that to her daughter, because if her daughter heard her say she wasn't thin enough to go on this trip, that her daughter would grow up saying the same kind of thing about herself.*

I remember once my sisters and I were visiting our parents, and we were driving home from dinner. My mother started talking about how beautiful and talented my two sisters were, and she kept going on about them. One of my sisters said, "What about Louise, Mom?" And my mother just kept shaking her head as if to say, "Well, what about her?" And I knew it was because I'm not thin like her other children, so I couldn't possibly have any special talents. I can't imagine doing that to my children.

WCG: *Do you think that she uses the whole weight issue— making fun of large people, pointing, staring, etc.—as a shield to protect herself from dealing with her own alcoholism?*

Louise: *Definitely. It strengthens her in a way, I think. It's so much easier for her to point out everyone else's problems, rather than deal with her own.*

WCG: *Your mother's thin, isn't she?*

Louise: *Yes. She's had six kids, and she's thin.*

WCG: *Does she like to point that out?*

Louise: *Yes, also that she exercised after she had her kids.*

WCG: But she doesn't sound like she's the least bit happy.

Louise: Oh, no. She's an alcoholic.

WCG: It's ironic, don't you think, that your mother is the thin
        woman, and certainly doesn't sound as if she's leading a
        life anyone would envy, while you're the "bad" daughter
        who won't get thin, and you sound like you're having a
        happy life.

Louise: (Laughs) You're right. That's a good point. I'll have to
        remember that one.

WCG: I think we've been brainwashed to believe that a thin
        woman automatically has a good life, but all you have to
        do is really take a good look around to realize that that's
        not true.

Louise: I know thin women who are fanatics about exercising to
        the point where it consumes their lives, where they don't
        have lives, really. It's very sad, the way they spend all
        their time at the gym. One of the other hairdressers I
        work with has a male customer who's a great-looking guy
        and the nicest man she ever met. His wife was a real
        fanatic about exercising and staying thin, and she was
        constantly putting him on a diet, making him get on the
        scale to be weighed, to the point where they finally
        ended up getting divorced because she didn't want to be
        married to him anymore. I don't think that's much of a
        life.

WCG: It's hard to build a whole life around a body, even if it's a
        perfect body.

Louise: I remember once I was in a department store looking for
        a dress for my brother's wedding. So I'm in the dress
        department, which happened to run into the petite

section. I wandered into the petite section without realizing it, and the manager of that department walked up to me and said, right to my face and as fast as she could, "YOU'RE IN THE PETITES," loud and clear as if she were announcing it. For all she knew, I could have been shopping for one of the petite women I know, but she was giving me my warning that I'd wandered off into the wrong department.

WCG: *Call 911.*

Louise: *I know. People get so weird when it comes to weight.*

WCG: *Fortunately, it doesn't sound like being heavy has gotten in the way of your doing what you wanted with your life. Louise: I don't think it has. I think I've got too much of a rebellious streak to let it stop me.*

I'm coming around to a way of thinking where I realize that my whole life I've been struggling and striving for my parents' approval. I've come to a point where I love myself, and the only person I need to prove anything to is myself. As long as I'm a good person, and I'm not doing anything to hurt anyone else, I should not constantly have to be proving myself. And I am a good person. I pay my bills, I go to work, I take care of my kids and I take care of them very well, the dinner is always on the table, and I'm faithful to my husband and faithful to myself, so what do I have to prove?

Ground Zero:
A Free Woman is Not a Number

Not too long ago, the ideal dress size for a woman was a 10; now it's a 6. Nancy Reagan wore a size 4 in her White House days and was considered fashionable. Has anyone noticed that this is a mere two sizes away from a size zero? As a metaphor for the direction American culture has taken, a direction which drives women to come as close as possible to disappearing, this scenario takes the cake, so to speak. Will American women finally wake up and realize they've been sold a bill of goods?

The impossible expectations which American society places upon women bring to mind the manipulations of abusive parents for whom nothing is ever good enough, who hold their children in thrall by never being satisfied with any effort or accomplishment. No doubt this is part of the reason why the only women judged as too thin are those who are visibly ill or actually dying of an eating disorder. Just as consistently high grades in school or stiflingly angelic behavior may be insufficient to elicit parental love and acceptance when we're young, later in life it becomes those 10, 20, 30 or more pounds lost which are still never enough to please those people (and society in general) who are only too happy to pick up where one's punitive parents left off.

As a result, those women who are not desperately striving for the nearest thing to literal invisibility have been turned into social, sexual, and political zeros by a culture that dictates exorbitant penalties for the failure or refusal to conform. Want to be seen as beautiful? Get thin and stay thin. Want your civil rights? Get thin and stay thin. Want a decent standard of medical care without lectures or ridicule? Get thin and stay thin. Want the benefit of the doubt? Get thin and stay thin. Want equal opportunity? Get thin and stay thin— or else. Again I ask, is this freedom?

When I began writing this book, I thought I was promoting an extremely radical point of view. Fat women healthy? Impossible! Fat women attractive? Absurd! Fat women entitled to social justice and common courtesy? Outrageous! Now, though, at the end, I realize that my arguments actually represent the middle ground. It is only because weight prejudice has become so overheated and irrational, so firmly established as a staple of American culture, that any line of reasoning which takes so much as one step back from this obsession seems, by comparison, militant. Also, as weight prejudice becomes more entrenched, so, too, does it become more inclusive; and millions of American women have learned the hard way that they need only be a mere 10 or 20 pounds "overweight" to feel its punitive, self-righteous sting.

A radical change is required in the way women relate to food in particular and to pleasure and entitlement in general. We must stop regarding the gratification derived from food as shameful or as a pathetic substitute for the "real" pleasures of sex. This is not to say that I think everyone should eat ice cream with every meal; simply that we should approach food without our breaths held in fear that we might experience too much of the "wrong" kind of pleasure. Everyone, not just thin people, deserves to experience the superb enjoyment that food can provide.

After all, considering the incalculable time and energy many women spend providing financially and/or emotionally for others, why aren't they entitled to give themselves some gratification? When is it their turn to be nourished, and why shouldn't they accomplish this themselves if no one else is willing or able? Instead, women are persuaded that being consumed by the needs of employers, men, and/or children is a validation of their femininity, while continual self-deprivation, anxiety, and guilt about food mean "caring about themselves." What's more disturbing about this line of thinking is its underlying rigid defensiveness, its brittle, macho insistence that the purely human need for comfort, whether achieved through food, physical contact, emotional release, or someone to talk with, is a sign of weakness and personal failure. Our puritanical culture has made the very concept of comfort vaguely suspect unless it comes in the limited forms approved by society, and eating for pleasure is especially condemned.

The fat woman is likewise condemned for her presumed hedonism, but she must refuse to fall prey to cultural typecasting. She must remember that there is often a yawning abyss between the image other people would force upon her and the reality of her existence. She must realize that if she does fit part or all of the description society draws of her, it may be because she has unwittingly lived down to expectations, especially if she has been surrounded since childhood by believers in the cliches, platitudes, and stereotypes of weight prejudice. She must insist upon being seen as more than just the poor lonely girl whom no one wants or the self-hating loser who has no control, no initiative, no style, and no dignity. Those who have carved out successful lives full of friendship and love must take every opportunity to stand up and be counted; and those who are just beginning to cast off the dismal image imposed upon them must resist the ignorance and intolerance of those who would halt that progress. Big women must not permit a world obsessed with reducing them one way or another to silent ghosts, to hold them to a different standard of accomplishment or to hold them up as peculiar failures.

As for me, I still don't have all the answers, but I know a few things. I know that active weight bigots dump their own miseries on the fat woman's back in the futile hope that if they just point and stare long enough and laugh loud enough, their scapegoat will disappear from sight and take everyone's problems and pain away with her. I know that passive weight bigots may actually give lip service to the idea that fat people are as good as everyone else, but ultimately they are unable or unwilling to accept that large and small individuals alike can be healthy, happy, and attractive. Most of all, I know that the path to freedom begins with not believing any of them, and being absolutely certain that they are wrong, not only in your head but all the way down in the center of your gut. So go ahead, get angry if you want. I promise not to tell you to tolerate, even excuse, your abusers because they're anxious or unhappy with themselves. Sometimes it seems that anger in a woman is considered an even greater sin than being fat; and while I'd be the last person to say that rage is an appropriate lifelong companion, it can be a gorgeous liberator. It can give you the strength to say, "Enough!"

I am a fat woman. I have struggled for years to reclaim the joy of living, the self-confidence, and the capacity to hope and dream that were stolen from me in my childhood and youth. I have worked long and hard to overcome my anger and fears. Although I've missed out on much that life has to offer, I refuse to waste another minute grieving for my past if I can possibly help it.

Still, when I pick up the paper and read an essay by a woman who complains that she cannot eat "with abandon" as she did when she was young and effortlessly slender, who revels in memories of "pack(ing) away...melted ice cream soup...(A) thousand Oreos, burgers, malts and candy" (Frank, 1992), I get angry all over again, thinking of society's smug lie that only fat women feast on such foods while thin girls nibble daintily at salads like fastidious rabbits. I still hesitate to get deeply involved in a world where it seems that men are not required to mature to a point where they value women as people instead of status symbols or servants, and where women are not allowed to mature to a point where they are strong enough to reject and overthrow such a system.

I see myself as a passionate and formidable woman with appetites for which I will make no apologies. I do not regard these appetites as neurotic, sickly weaknesses to be stamped out, but rather as intense confirmation that I am alive. I will not camouflage my body with dark, drab clothes or by hiding indoors. I will abide no insinuations that I am only a true woman if my hips and thighs grow smaller and my breasts larger. I will never willingly be a human sacrifice to the insecurities of a pack of grown-up schoolyard bullies. I mean to have my freedom and *eat* it, too.

Weight bigotry is a sad prejudice. Unless we hold fast and refuse to cave in to its pressures, it tends to creep up on us, one day, one insult, one injustice at a time, until the moment comes when we realize we're either walking through life with our head down or seething with a volcanic, suppressed rage which society arrogantly attributes to our own so-called failures. Ironically, the very banality of weight prejudice raises a deadly serious question; namely, if people insist on harassing, humiliating, and exploiting others for something as trivial as weight, what hope do we have of ever overcoming the much older and even more virulent prejudices based on race, gender, and religion?

Despite all the rhetoric back and forth, political correctness (when it is not condemning some prejudices and endorsing others simultaneously) is at its best when it calls for an end to snap judgments and a social hierarchy based on hackneyed stereotypes. It is an attempt to carve a level playing field out of a morass of social entitlements and deprivations based on class, a prospect that is not only frightening in that it brings chaos to the order that lies in assumptions and prejudgments, but also exhausting in the complexity it represents. Such an outlook makes it impossible for us to tell who's good or bad, trustworthy or suspicious, lovable or repellent, based on gender or race or religion—or body size. It forces us to give everyone the benefit of the doubt, to come to terms with the fact that despite our most strenuous efforts, life is deliciously and uncomfortably complicated. It's certainly not the easiest way to live, but it's infinitely preferable to seeing the final verdict in people's eyes before you can even say hello; and it's a lot more interesting than making up your own mind about people before you've even met them.

The time has come when big women must stop asking ourselves if a man-made modern world deliberately designed only for the lean and mean will ever accept *us* as we are, and instead ask whether or not *we,* the invisible women of America, should continue to tolerate a bigoted and literally narrow-minded society that claims to know our bodies and minds better than we ourselves ever could. We must each decide if the price of freedom is one we're willing to pay. Most importantly, we must hold up our heads and turn our backs on the maniacal cult of anorexic chic that has shadowed so many hearts and killed so much joy. We have nothing to lose but the chains of our invisibility.

> *No woman can call herself free who does not own and control her body.*
>   Margaret Sanger

Resources

Association for the Health Enrichment of Large People
AHELP
P.O. Drawer C
Radford, VA 24143
703/731-1778 (phone or fax)
Joe McVoy, PhD., Director
Group for professionals who use the non-dieting approach.
Newsletter. AHELP forum.

Council on Size & Weight Discrimination, Inc.
P.O. Box 305
Mt. Marion, NY 12456
914/679-1209 Fax: 914/679-1206
Miriam Berg, President
Anti-size-discrimination activist group. Influences public opinion and policy through education, information, and networking. (International No Diet Coalition is a partially funded project of this council.)

Gürze Books
P.O. Box 2238
Carlsbad, CA 92018
800/756-7533 Fax: 619/434-5476
Lindsey Hall and Leigh Cohn, Owners
Publishes and distributes a variety of books on eating disorders, body image, size acceptance, and related issues for lay and professional readers. Quarterly journal, bi-monthly newsletter. Free catalogue on request.

Largesse: The Network for Size Esteem
   P.O. Box 9404
   New Haven, CT   06534-0404
   203/787-1624 (phone or fax)
Karen W. and Richard K. Stimson, Co-directors
International resource and information clearinghouse for
size diversity empowerment. Database, archives, support
material, quarterly newsletter, *Food for Thought*, and bi-
monthly bulletin, *Size Esteem*.

National Association to Advance Fat Acceptance, Inc.
   NAAFA
   P.O. Box 188620
   Sacramento, CA 95818
   916/558-6880 Fax: 916/558–6881
Sally E. Smith, Executive Director
National organization working to end discrimination and
empower fat people through education, advocacy and
member support. Bi-monthly *NAAFA Newsletter*, pamphlets,
annual convention, and regional events. Over 50 chapters in
the US and Canada.

Bibliography

Grateful appreciation is given to all publishers for allowing me to use copyrighted material, as noted within this bibliography. Two of my local newspapers were also generous in allowing me to reprint quotations:

Adam P: *Art of the Third Reich*. New York, Harry N. Abrams, Inc., 1992, pp. 110, 188, 200, 252. All rights reserved.

Adam R: *A Woman's Place* (1910-1975). New York, W.W. Norton & Company, 1975, p. 32.

Alman I: Ask Isadora. *Bay Area Guardian*, July 15, 1992, p. 24.

Allport G: *The Nature of Prejudice*. New York, Doubleday & Company, Inc., 1958, p. 317.

Alt C: Vicki Lawrence talk show, May 13, 1994.

Anonymous: Letter to the Editor, *BBW* magazine. October 1990, p. 66.

Arky R, Davidson C, Weld F: 1995 *Physicians' Desk Reference*. Montvale, NJ, Medical Economics Data Production Company, pp. 944, 945.

Asimov N: Many Innovations, But No Solutions. *San Francisco Chronicle*, May 26, 1993, p. A9.

Associated Press, Washington: Big Guys Tell Kids to Shape Up. Printed in *San Francisco Chronicle*, May 2, 1991, p. A2.

Associated Press: Survey Reveals Ignorance About Sexual Diseases. Printed in *San Francisco Chronicle*, February 14, 1995, p. A3.

Associated Press: High court mulling rights of fat people. *San Francisco Examiner*, June 20, 1993, p. 1, *et seq*.

Associated Press: Navy petty officer faces discharge for being 12 pounds overweight. *San Francisco Examiner*, June 13, 1993, p. B-5.

Bailey B: Shredded records muddle doctor case. *San Jose Mercury News*, August 5, 1991, p. 1B.

Bailey J: She might have inherited millions, but for her mother. *Wall Street Journal*, November 25, 1991, p. A1, *et seq*.

Barnum A: Insurers Use Genes to Deny Coverage. *San Francisco Chronicle*, December 2, 1992, p. 1/A8.

Bennett W, Gurin J: *The Dieter's Dilemma*. New York, Basic Books, Inc., 1982, pp. 4, 5.

Berg D: The Lighter Side of Hang-Ups. *Mad Magazine*, October 1972, p. 34.

Berland T. *Consumer Guide: Rating The Diets*. Skokie, IL, 1974a, pp. 33, 83-84, 87, 93, 94.

Berland T: *The Dieter's Almanac*. New York, World Almanac Publications, 1984b, pp. 143, 158, 159.

Blickenstorfer C: Survey of Male Fat Admirers. *The NAAFA Workbook*. Sacramento, CA, pp. 5-7.

Blum D: Studies on beauty raise a number of ugly findings. *San Francisco Examiner*, February 16, 1992.

Bockar J: *The Last Best Diet Book*. New York, Stein and Day, 1980, pp. 14, 30-31, 32, 41, 42, 45, 60, 141, 146, 195, 197.

Bordo S: *Body/Politics: Women and the Discourses of Science*. Jacobus, Keller, and Shuttleworth eds., New York, Routledge, Chapman and Hall, Inc., 1990, pp. 100, 105.

Boston Women's Health Book Collective: *The New Our Bodies, Ourselves*. New York, Simon & Schuster, 1984, pp. 22, 187.

Boulware J: Slap Shots. *San Francisco Weekly*, February 8, 1995, p. 20.

Bouvier L, Grant L: *How Many Americans? Population, Immigration and the Environment*. San Francisco, Sierra Club Books, 1994, p. 105, n.10.

Brady J: In Step With: Jean Marsh. *Parade* magazine, July 12, 1992, p. 14.

Broun H, Britt G: *Christians Only*. The Vanguard Press, 1931, pp. 15, 224-25; Da Capo Press, 1974.

Bruno F: *Born To Be Slim*. New York, Harper & Row, 1978, pp. 83, 87.

Buber M: *The Knowledge of Man* ed. M. Friedman; trans. Robert Gregor Smith. Harper & Row, George Allen & Unwin Ltd., 1965; quoted from *The Enduring Questions*, by Melvin Rader, New York, Holt, Rinehard & Winston, 1969, p. 658.

Burke C: The Trail to Tailhook. This World, *San Francisco Chronicle*, August 16, 1992, p. 7; originally printed in *The New Republic*.

Canada W: *Beauty Surgery*. Cosmetic Surgery of Las Vegas, no date of publication or copyright noted, p. 118.

Carey A: Losing weight for bathing-suit season. *San Jose Mercury News*, June 16, 1993, p. 6E.

Carlisle B: Personals, by Leah Garchik, *San Francisco Chronicle*, January 7, 1992, p. D1.

Carroll J: Staying On Top Of It All. *San Francisco Chronicle*, November 6, 1992, p. D3.

CBS: Eye to Eye. January 5, 1995.

Chapian M, Coyle N: *Free To Be Thin*. Minneapolis, MN, Bethany House, 1979, p. 175.

Cheers 'n' Jeers: *TV Guide*, January 11, 1995, p. 23.

Chernin K: *The Obsession: Reflections on the Tyranny of Slenderness*. New York, Harper & Row, 1981, pp. 4-7.

Chicago Tribune/New York Times: The Slimming of America. *San Jose Mercury News*, December 5, 1994, p. 4A.

Chronicle Wire Services: Farrakhan, Former Aide Renews Attacks Against Whites, Jews. *San Francisco Chronicle*, February 28, 1994, p. A11.

Chutkow P: The Peasant King. Datebook, *San Francisco Chronicle*, April 24, 1994, p. 30.

Cimons M: New attitude urged toward obesity. *San Jose Mercury News*, December 6, 1994, p. 6A.

Cordell F, Giebler G: *Psychological War On Fat*. Niles, IL, Argus Communications, 1977, p. 34.

Cowley G, Hager M: Sleeping With the Enemy. *Newsweek*, December 9, 1991, p. 58.

Diebel D: *Finding Mr. Right: A Woman's Guide to Meeting Men*. Houston, TX, Gemini publishing, 1990, p. 128.

Driscoll A: Inhaler scrutinized in mystery death. *San Jose Mercury News*, July 5, 1995, p. 7A.

Dowling C: *Perfect Women*. New York, Summit Books, 1988, pp. 103-104.

Dream On: June 13, 1992.

Drozdiak W: France May Ban Test-Tube Babies For Older Women. *San Francisco Chronicle*, January 4, 1994, p. 1.

Eades M: *Thin So Fast*. New York, Warner Books, 1989, p. 14.

Eckert SC: The Unkindest Cut of All. *NAAFA Newsletter*, December 1992, p. 4.

Edell D: Dr. Dean Edell Medical Journal, *San Francisco Chronicle*, December 31, 1992, p. D4.

Edelstein B: *The Woman Doctor's Diet for Women*. New York, Ballantine Books, New York, 1977, pp. 6, 42, 43, 66, 112.

Esquer M: AIDS Message Fails In Hispanic Communities. Open Forum, *San Francisco Chronicle*, 1992.

Fay M: Book review of *The Rise of Life on Earth* by Joyce Carol Oates, *Express Newspaper*, October 1991, p. 18.

Fernandez E: Health: The wages of sin. *San Francisco Examiner*, November 14, 1993, p. A12.

Finke N: Actress Is Weighed Down By Hollywood Attitudes. Sunday Datebook, *San Francisco Chronicle*, February 17, 1991, pp. 33-34.

Firestone S: *The Dialectic of Sex: The Case for Feminist Revolution*. New York, Bantam Books, 1970, p. 152.

Fox M: Good Grief: Playfulness Fuels Tale of Death. Sunday Datebook, *San Francisco Chronicle*, April 26, 1992, p. 48.

Frank J: Eat It And Weep. *San Francisco Chronicle*, September 6, 1992, p. 16.

Fraser L: The Overweight Want Their Rights. *Working Woman Magazine*; reprinted in *San Francisco Chronicle*, June 22, 1994, p. E7.

Garchik L: Personals. *San Francisco Chronicle*, May 22, 1991, p. A8.

Gierlichs P (ed.): *The Nazi Primer: Official Handbook for Schooling the Hitler Youth*. Fritz Brennecke (Herausgeber); 1937, pp. xx.

Gold A, Briller S: *Diet Watchers Guide*. New York, Grosset & Dunlap, 1968, pp. 11, 22.

Goodman E: Beauty Queens And Platforms. *Boston Globe* (reprinted in *San Francisco Chronicle*), September 23, 1993, p. A25.

Gortmaker S, Must A, Perrin J, Sobol A, Dietz W: Social and Economic Consequences of Overweight in Adolescence and Young Adulthood. *The New England Journal of Medicine*, September 30, 1993, p. 1011.

Gransden G: From Russia, With Love. *Los Angeles Times*, August 15, 1991, p. E1.

Grapevine: A Dead-End Street. *TV Guide*, August 1, 1992, p. 4.

Guisewite C: Cathy comic strip, May 26, 1991. Guralnik D, Ed.: *Webster's New World Dictionary of the American Language*, Second College Edition, New York, World Publishing, 1972, p. 982.

Gurley Brown H: *Having It All*. New York, Simon & Schuster, 1982, pp. 71, 74, 98.

Gustafson N: *Lifetime Weight Control*. La Mesa, CA, Western Schools Press, 1988a, pp. 2-13 to 2-14.

Gustafson N: *Lifetime Weight Control Patient Counseling*, 3rd ed. La Mesa, CA, Western Schools Press, 1993b, p. 30.

Guthmann E: Altman's 'Player' for the 90's. *San Francisco Chronicle*, April 23, 1992a, p. E2.

Guthmann E: Midnight Movie 'Gross Out' Just Plain Disgusting. *San Francisco Chronicle*, February 15, 1992b, p. C7.

Hampson R: Ex-Wives Trash Hubbies. *San Francisco Chronicle*, May 18, 1992, p. B3.

Haney D: 'Yo-yo' Diets Called Heavy Heart Risk. *San Francisco Examiner*, June 26, 1991, pp. 1, A12.

Harvey D: How Good Germans Turned Into Nazis. Sunday Datebook, *San Francisco Chronicle*, November 3, 1991, p. 32.

Hauler J: Responses to 'Can't Accept Fat.' Letter to *Radiance* magazine, Fall 1991, p. 4.

Heller K: Unplanned Parenthood. *San Jose Mercury News*, March 14, 1993, p. 1L.

Heller R, Heller R: *The Carbohydrate Addict's Diet*. New York, Dutton, 1991, p. 18.

Herrin A: Weighty questions. *San Jose Mercury News*, September 4, 1991, p. 1D.

Hillel M, Henry C: *Of Pure Blood*. New York, McGraw-Hill, Inc., 1976, pp. 47-48, 103. Reproduced with permission of McGraw-Hill, Inc.

Hughes R: A Sampler of Witless Truisms. *Time* magazine, July 30, 1990, p. 66.

Jablonski M: The Cutting Edge. *NAAFA Newsletter*, Nov. 1993, p. 3.

Jacobs J: Elephant Seals. *West Magazine*, October 27, 1991, p. 4.

Johnston T: Letter to the Editor. *San Francisco Examiner*, January 1992.

Joslyn L: October 21, 1992 letter sent by Weight Watchers to employers advertising its At Work diet program; signed by Laura Joslyn, Executive Assistant to the Vice President, Weight Watchers of Central Florida; Weight Watchers of Northern Alabama.

Kahn A: Dire Images of Beauty, *San Francisco Chronicle*, June 6, 1991a, p. B3.

Kahn A: Sex, Lies and More Lies. *San Francisco Chronicle*, April 15, 1992b, p. B4.

Kahn A: The Women of the Night. *San Francisco Chronicle*, June 17, 1991c, p. D3.

Kaplan L: *Adolescence: The Farewell to Childhood*. New York, Simon and Schuster, 1984, p. 116.

Kato D: The Single File: Bachelors. They're Out There, and They Say They're Interested In—Eventually—Settling Down. What Do They Value in a Woman? Listen While They Tell Us. *San Jose Mercury News*, September 15, 1991, p. 6L.

Kaufman J, Wolfe S, *et al.*: *Over The Counter Pills That Don't Work.* Washington, DC, Public Citizen Health Research Group, 1983, pp. 81-82.

Kevles D: In *The Name of Eugenics*. Berkeley, California, University of California Press, 1985, p. 139.

Kitaen T: Grapevine, *TV Guide*. September 5, 1992, p. 2.

Krajick K: Private Passions & Public Health. *Psychology Today*, May 1988, p. 56.

Krogh D: *Smoking: The Artificial Passion*. W.H. Freeman and Co., 1991; quoted in *San Francisco Chronicle*, Female Smokers Rivaling Men, by Claudia Morain, July 11, 1994, p. E7.

Kushner H: *When Bad Things Happen to Good People*. New York, Avon Books, 1983, p. 120.

Lampert L: Fat Like Me. *Ladies' Home Journal*, May 1993, p. 215.

Landers A: *San Jose Mercury News*, February 27, 1992a, p. 5D.

Landers A: *San Jose Mercury News*. July 7, 1993b, p. 2D.

Landers A: *San Francisco Examiner*, August 29, 1993c, p. D-6.

Lara A: Souls Don't Gain Weight; People Do. *San Francisco Chronicle*, 1991, p. E8.

Lattin D: Secret files on Americans' Genes. *San Francisco Chronicle*, February 17, 1992, p. 1.

Leary W: Exercise May Work as Well In Small Doses, U.S. Report Says. *New York Times*, reprinted in *San Francisco Chronicle*, July 30, 1993, p. A19.

Lee Harris A: Americans should give good beef its due. *San Francisco Chronicle*, p. 8.

LeShan E: *Winning the Losing Battle*. New York, Thomas Y. Crowell Publishers, 1979, pp. 5, 12.

Logan M: Santa Barbara's Lucky Cinderfella. *TV Guide*, December 14, 1991, p. 24.

Love C: People in the News. *San Jose Mercury News*, May 18, 1995, p. 4A.

Lucas G: Smoking Foes to Sue Wilson. *San Francisco Chronicle*, February 21, 1992, p. A21.

Lyons P: Fitness, Feminism and the Health of Fat Women. From *Overcoming Fear of Fat*, New York, Harrington Park Press, 1989, p. 74. Reprinted by permission.

Marine C: Undying Love. *Image Magazine*, June 23, 1991, p. 18, *et seq*.

Married With Children: October 25, 1991.

Marshall J: Looks Count, Says Study on Earning Power. *San Francisco Chronicle*, November 1, 1993, p. A13.

Martin J: Dear Miss Manners; November 13, 1991a, *San Francisco Chronicle*, p. B4.

Martin J: Dear Miss Manners. *San Francisco Chronicle*, January 31, 1992b, p. D5.

Maurstad T: For all that talk, romance game shows betray their innocence. *Dallas Morning News*, printed in *San Jose Mercury News*, July 3, 1992, p. 3E.

McAllister Smart J: The Gender Gap. *Vegetarian Times*, February 1995, p. 80.

McDougal D: New 'L.A. Law' character: Is she the real item—or not? *San Jose Mercury News*, December 9, 1991, pp. 1C, 4C.

Miller M: Safety and Long-Term Effectiveness of Diet Drugs Are Still Uncertain. *Wall Street Journal*, July 20, 1994, p. A6.

Miller R: Don't expect any good, clean fun from 'Maid.' *San Jose Mercury News*, January 13, 1992, p. 10B.

Millman M: *Such A Pretty Face: Being Fat In America*. New York, Berkeley Books, 1980, pp. 77, 158, 205.

Milstead J: Fat Like Her. *Big Beautiful Woman* magazine, April, 1994, pp. 19-20.

Minton L: What it feels like to be fat: Readers speak out. Lisa Ames; Tracy Elkus. Fresh Voices, *Parade* magazine, April 26, 1992, p. 24.

Mirkin G with Foreman L: *Getting Thin: All About Fat—How You Get It, How You Lose It, How You Keep It Off For Good*. Boston, MA, Little, Brown and Company, 1983, pp. 149-150.

Mitchard J: And Now Meet the Rest of TV's Unlikely Heartthrobs. *TV Guide*, January 8, 1994, pp. 14, 15.

Morgan E: *The Descent of Woman*. New York, Stein and Day, 1972, p. 229.

Morris D: *The Human Zoo*. London, Corgi Books, 1971; pp. 75, 85, 87, 88, 89, 90, 101, 102, 108.

Mosse G, ed.: *Nazi Culture*. New York, Grosset & Dunlap, 1966, pp. 64-65. [From Hans F.K. Gunther, *Kleine Rassenkunde des Deutschen Volkes* (Munich, 1929), pp. 9-13, 21-25, 59. (This extract has been taken from the 1933 edition.)]

Murphy M, Swertlow F: Delta Redesigned. *TV Guide*, July 4, 1992, p. 10.

NAAFA Workbook: Results of the NAAFA Survey on Employment Discrimination. Summary abstracted from a survey and article by Esther Rothblum, Pamela Brand, Carol Miller, and Helen Oetjen at the University of Vermont). *NAAFA Workbook*, pp. 6-13.

NAAFA Workbook: "News Roundup," January/February 1992,pp. 6-13. All *NAAFA Workbook* quotes reprinted with permission from: NAAFA Inc., PO Box 188620, Sacramento, CA 95818; 916/558-6880.

Nachman G: Time to Toss Out Some Unaired Opinions. Datebook, *San Francisco Chronicle*, May 10, 1992, p. 17.

Nemetz JC: *Better Than Ever*. No publisher indicated, 1988, p. 97.

Nevius CW: Life's a Beach—Just Barely. *San Francisco Chronicle*, July 28, 1992, p. E5.

New York Times: Bad Marriage, Double Slaying and a Hung Jury. Reported in *San Francisco Chronicle*, September 23, 1991, p. D3 *et seq*.

Obituary, *San Francisco Chronicle*, May 9, 1991.

Oliver MF, Kurien VA, Greenwood TW: Relation Between Serum-Free Fatty Acids and Arrhythmias and Death after Acute Myocardial Infarction. *Lancet*, April 6, 1968, pp. 710-714. Quoted from Berland, T: *Consumer Guide: Rating The Diets*. Skokie, IL, Publications International, Ltd., 1974a, p. 254.

Orbach S: *Fat Is A Feminist Issue*. New York, Berkeley Medallion/New York, Paddington Press, 1978, pp. 31, 35.

Orr J: Twelve Bars and a Turnaround. *West Magazine, San Jose Mercury News*, July 19, 1992, p. 18.

Parker J: The Role of Stigmatization in Fat People's Avoidance of Physical Exercise. From *Overcoming Fear of Fat*, New York, Harrington Park Press, 1989, pp. 56-57. Reprinted by permission.

Phibbs C: Letter to the Editor. *San Francisco Examiner*, September 18, 1994.

Plaskin G: Liz Taylor's Renaissance. *San Francisco Chronicle*, January 7, 1992, p. D4.

Pois R: *National Socialism and the Religion of Nature*. New York, St. Martin's Press, 1986, pp. 125-26.

Privitere A: Jobs Threatened By 'Lifestyle Discrimination', Reuter, *San Francisco Examiner*, July 21, 1991, p. A5.

Proctor R: *Racial Hygiene: Medicine Under the Nazis*, Cambridge, MA, Harvard University Press, copyright 1988 by the President and Fellows of Harvard College, pp. 56, 103-104, 194-195, 195-196, 197. Reprinted by permission.

Quindlen A: What Really Counts In Thin Air. May 18, 1993, *San Francisco Chronicle*, p. A16.

Rader D: The Day The Acting Bug Bit Me. *Parade* magazine, May 3, 1992, p. 24.

Ragel J: No-Sweat Style. *TV Guide*, May 28, 1994, p. 16.

Ratner D: Santa Cruz Gives Tentative OK To Law on Personal Appearance. *San Francisco Chronicle*, January 15, 1992, p. 1 *et seq*.

Recreation & Community Services Brochure. City of Albany, Fall 1991, p. 12.

Rensin D: The Cop You Hate to Love. *TV Guide*, March 5, 1994, p. 13.

Reuters: Americans Still Kind of Porky. *San Francisco Chronicle*, February 22, 1992, p. C1.

Rivera R: Letter to the editor. *San Francisco Chronicle*, December 13, 1991, p. A34.

Rives D: *Walk Yourself Thin*. Ventura, CA, Moon River Publishing, 1990, pp. 8, 63, 103-104, 153-54. Reprinted by permission.

Roberts S, Staver P: Why American Children Are in Such Bad Shape. *American Health Magazine*, reprinted in *San Francisco Chronicle*, October 27, 1992, p. D3.

Roemer J, Cothran G, Clark K: Eat your words. *San Francisco Weekly*, February 24, 1993, p. 7.

Rubenstein C: Food, Not Sex, Is New Sin of Choice. American Health Magazine Service (printed in *San Francisco Chronicle*, January 4, 1992, p. C1).

Rubin T: *Anti-Semitism: A Disease of the Mind*. New York, Continuum, 1990c, p. 29.

Rubin T: *Forever Thin*. New York, Gramercy, 1970a, pp. 70, 93, 106.

Rubin T: *The Thin Book by a Formerly Fat Psychiatrist*. New York, Pinnacle Books, 1972b, p. 12. Quoted from Berland, T: *Consumer Guide: Rating The Diets*. Skokie, IL, Publications International, Ltd., 1974a, p. 33.

Lord Russell of Liverpool: *The Scourge of the Swastika*. New York, Ballantine Books, 1954, pp. 182, 216-217.

Russo F: The Grunt-and-Sweat Fitness Date. *San Francisco Chronicle*, November 24, 1991, p. 2.

Sacker I and Zimmer M: *Dying to be Thin*. New York, Warner Books, 1987, pg. 32.

San Francisco Chronicle. A Fat Chance (editorial). October 31, 1991, p. A20.

Sanger M: *Parade* magazine, December 1, 1963.

Sapolsky R: *Why Don't Zebras Get Ulcers?* New York, W.H. Freeman and Company, 1994, pp. 65, 122, 151

Sartre J: *Anti-Semite and Jew*. New York, Schocken Books, trans. by George J. Becker, 1948, pp. 26, 34.

Savage D: Savage Love. *San Francisco Weekly*, July 6, 1994, p. 48. Reprinted by permission.

Schiff M: *Doctor Schiff's Miracle Weight-Loss Guide*. New York, Parker Publishing Company, Inc., 1974, pp. 38-40, 72, 73, 156, 202-203, 216.

Schrage M: Enlisting technology to battle fat. *San Francisco Examiner*, September 29, 1991, p. E-3.

Schroeder C: *Fat Is Not A Four-Letter Word*. Minneapolis, MN, Chronimed Publishing, 1992, pp. 97, 101-102, 117, 137, 140-143, 159-160. Reprinted with permission from CHRONIMED Publishing.

Schulz C: *Nobody's Perfect, Charlie Brown*. Greenwich, CT, Fawcett Publications, Inc., 1969.

Scott N: A libel written in blood. Review of *The Blood Libel Legend—A Casebook in Anti-Semitic Folklore* by Alan Dundes; *San Francisco Examiner*, February 16, 1992, p. D-5.

Selvin J: Ann Peebles Redeems Her Rain Check. Sunday Datebook, *San Francisco Chronicle*, April 26, 1992, p. 51.

Shakespeare W: *The Merchant of Venice*. New York, New American Library, 1965, p. 87.

Shales T: 'L.A. Law' A Riot of Mediocrity. *Washington Post*, reprinted in *San Francisco Chronicle*, October 22, 1992, p. E1.

Shapiro S: Sheer Delight, Sheer Agony, *Avenue* Magazine. Reprinted in *San Francisco Chronicle*, June 3, 1992, p. D5.

Shaw C: Notes from a speech by Susan Wooley, Ph.D.: Obesity Treatment Today: Broken Promises and Lost Opportunity: *BBW* magazine, November 1991, p. 35.

Sjoo M, Mor B: *The Great Cosmic Mother: Rediscovering the Religion of the Earth.* San Francisco, Harper & Row, 1987, p. 68.

Simmons R: *Never-Say-Diet.* New York, Warner Books, 1980, pp. 16-17, 36, 37, 76, back cover.

Smith L: Gossip. *San Francisco Chronicle*, July 31, 1991, p. E1.

Smith S: In Memoriam. *NAAFA Newsletter*, October 1992, p. 6.

Spock B: Decent and Indecent. Quoted in *Sisterhood Is Powerful*, ed. by Robin Morgan, New York, Random House, 1970, pp. 35-36.

Squire S: *The Slender Balance: Causes and Cures for Bulimia, Anorexia & the Weight-Loss/Weight-Gain Seesaw.* New York, G.P. Putnam's Sons, 1983, pp. 224-226.

Stack P: Chevy Chase Can't Fill Role of 'Man of the House.' *San Francisco Chronicle*, March 3, 1995, p. C6.

Starr Seibel D: Unholy Smokes. Datebook, *San Francisco Chronicle*, June 14, 1992, p. 43.

Stein R: Audrey Hepburn Remains a Class Act. *San Francisco Chronicle*, January 24, 1992, p. E3.

Steinberg M: *A Partisan Guide To The Jewish Problem.* New York, Charter Books, 1945, pp. 70, 71.

Steinem G: I'm Not The Woman In My Mind. *Parade* magazine, January 12, 1992, p. 10.

Stress and Fat. Health & Fitness News Service, reported in Obesity and Health (*San Francisco Chronicle*, October 25, 1993, p. E9).

Stuart R, Jacobson B: *Weight, Sex & Marriage: A Delicate Balance.* New York, W.W. Norton & Company, 1987, pp. 12, 26, 36.

Sumrall H: Paula Abdul—all glitter, no gold. *San Jose Mercury News*, December 16, 1991, p. 3C.

Taylor M: Innocence Lost. *This World*, June 7, 1992, p. 8, *et seq.*

Thomas M: New York *Observer*, as quoted in *San Francisco Chronicle* "Personals," March 11, 1994, p. C18.

Thum G, Thum M: *The Persuaders: Propaganda in War and Peace*, New York, Atheneum, 1972, pp. 170-71.

Trudeau G: Doonesbury comic strip. February 10, 1992.

TV Guide: Grapevine. May 23, 1992, p. 4.

TV Guide: Week of January 25, 1992, p. 101 [advertisement].

TV Update. *TV Guide*: Week of March 28, 1992, p. 32.

Twain, M: Consistency, 1887: from *Mark Twain's Speeches* by Albert Bigelow Paine, 1922, p. 130.

von Franz M: *Man and His Symbols*. New York, Doubleday, 1964, p. 224.

Wadden TA, Stunkard AJ: A controlled trial of very-low calorie diet, behavior therapy, and their combination in the treatment of obesity. *Journal of Consultations in Clinical Psychology*, 1986: quoted in *Lifetime Weight Control Patient Counseling*, p. 30, 3rd ed., by Nancy J. Gustafson, MS, LRD; Western Schools Press, 1993b.

Walker M: Beetle Bailey comic strip, January 12, 1992.

Warrick P: The Short Shelf Life of Models. *Los Angeles Times*, reported in the *San Francisco Chronicle*, August 10, 1992, p. D3.

Washington Post: Chicago Police Face Waist-Busting Plan, *Washington Post*, January 2, 1992, reprinted in *San Francisco Chronicle*, p. A7.

Welch D: *Propaganda and the German Cinema, 1933-1945*. Oxford, Clarendon Press, 1983, p. 121, 294.

Westin J: *The Thin Book*. Minneapolis, Minnesota, CompCare Publications, 1978, pp. 163, 168.

Wiebe J: *3500 Calories=One Pound*. Camano Island, WA, Wiebe Enterprises, Inc., 1980, p. 9.

Wilkinson S: "This shocking public display of flesh oughta' be banned." July 19, 1991, *Philadelphia Daily News*.

Williams R: Let Freedom Ring. *The NAAFA Workbook*, p. 4-1. Permission granted for reprinting article by Russell F. Williams per NAAFA Program Director Sharon McDonell.

Winokur S: The Human Condition. *Image* Magazine, Aug. 2, 1992, p. 12.

Wolf N: *The Beauty Myth*. New York, William Morrow and Company, Inc. 1991, pp. 146, 174, 187, 189.

Woodman M: *The Owl Was a Baker's Daughter: Obesity, Anorexia Nervosa and the Repressed Feminine*. Toronto, Canada, Inner City Books, 1980, pp. 7, 11, 40, 42, 57, 97.

Wyse L: *Blonde Beautiful Blonde: How to Look, Live, Work and Think Blonde*. New York, M. Evans and Company, Inc., 1980, pp. 37, 39, 118, 159, 160.

Zehme B: The Devil Makes Her Do It. Sunday Datebook, *San Francisco Chronicle*, May 3, 1992, p. 39.

Zeiger H: *The Case Against Adolph Eichmann*. New York, Penguin USA, 1960, pp. 20, 180, 181. Copyright 1960 by Henry Zeiger. Used by permission of Penguin USA.

Zerbe K: *The Body Betrayed*. Carlsbad, CA, Gürze Books, 1995, p. 305.

Zimmer D: "Diet Shows" Insulting and Unacceptable. *NAAFA Newsletter*, March 1992, p. 2.

Index

Order Form

The Invisible Woman is available at bookstores and libraries. Copies may also be ordered directly from Gürze Books.

FREE Catalogue

The Gürze Eating Disorders Bookshelf Catalogue has more than 80 books and tapes on eating disorders and related topics, including body image, size-acceptance, self-esteem, feminist issues, and more. It is a valuable resource that includes listings of non-profit associations, and it is handed out by therapists, educators, and other health care professionals throughout the world.

Please send me:

____ **FREE** copies of the *Gürze Eating Disorders Bookshelf Catalogue*

____ copies of *The Invisible Woman*
   $14.95 each (1-4 copies) plus $2.50 each for shipping and handling

____ copies of *The Invisible Woman*
   $11.95 each (5+ copies) plus $1.95 each for shipping and handling

Quantity discounts are available on large orders.

NAME _____

ADDRESS _____

CITY, ST, ZIP _____

PHONE _____

Mail a copy of this order form to:

Gürze Books (TIW)
P.O. Box 2238
Carlsbad, CA 92018
Order by phone: 800/756-7533